STRATEGIES FOR CREATING A TEAM-WINNING EFFORT

Mackie Shilstone's
Body Plan for Kids

MACKIE SHILSTONE

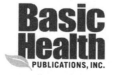

Basic Health
PUBLICATIONS, INC.

The information contained in this book is based upon the research and personal and professional experiences of the author. It is not intended as a substitute for consulting with your physician or other healthcare provider. Any attempt to diagnose and treat an illness should be done under the direction of a healthcare professional.

The publisher does not advocate the use of any particular healthcare protocol but believes the information in this book should be available to the public. The publisher and author are not responsible for any adverse effects or consequences resulting from the use of the suggestions, preparations, or procedures discussed in this book. Should the reader have any questions concerning the appropriateness of any procedures or preparation mentioned, the author and the publisher strongly suggest consulting a professional healthcare advisor.

Basic Health Publications, Inc.
28812 Top of the World Drive
Laguna Beach, CA 92651
949-715-7327 • www.basichealthpub.com

Library of Congress Cataloging-in-Publication Data

Shilstone, Mackie.
   Mackie Shilstone's body plan for kids / Mackie Shilstone.
     p. cm.
   Includes bibliographical references and index.
   ISBN 978-1-59120-249-3
  1. Physical fitness for children. 2. Exercise for children.
3. Diet therapy for children.
I. Title. II. Title: Body plan for kids.

   RJ133.S54 2009
   613.2083—dc22

                                                          2008055713

Copyright © 2009 by Mackie Shilstone.

Editor: Cheryl Hirsch
Typesetting/Graphic design: Gary A. Rosenberg
Cover design: Mike Stromberg

Printed in the United States of America

10   9   8   7   6   5   4   3   2   1

Contents

Acknowledgments

To my family—my wife, Sandy; my sons, Scott and Spencer; and the loving memory of my father, Cecil, and my mother, Frances—for all the support a husband, father, and son could ever ask for from his family.

To my writer, Dean M. Shapiro, for his continuing ability to strive for excellence, often in the face of adversity and my hard-driving, goal-oriented personality.

To my assistant, Michelle Hyde, for taking the pressure off me to let me be me.

To my team members at East Jefferson General Hospital in Metairie, Louisiana, for welcoming me to their family and for being a great team to house my program, The Fitness Principle with Mackie Shilstone.

To Dr. Michael Wasserman, my son's pediatrician, to Dr. Robert Gensure, pediatric endocrinologist, and to Dr. Rob Dahmes, a pediatric child psychiatrist, my deepest appreciation for their willingness to share their knowledge and their mutual desire to attack childhood obesity and its causes, and to share treatment options with readers of this book.

To Scott Johnson, my partner in five General Nutrition Centers (GNC) franchises and publisher of Basic Media, and to Norm Goldfind, publisher of Basic Health Publications, for their eagerness to publish this book.

To Cheryl Hirsch, our editor at Basic Health Publications, for her great job in editing the original manuscript, and for the finished product.

To Gary Rosenberg, typesetter and designer at Basic Health Publications, for creating a fun and effective book design.

To Julie Fortenberry, my nutritionist at The Fitness Principle at East Jefferson General Hospital, for her excellent work in designing the nutrition guidelines and sample meal plans for our readers, and for her valuable assistance in guiding us along on the final edit of the manuscript.

To the East Jefferson General Hospital Marketing Department for their invaluable help in development of many of the graphics used in this book.

To Cherry Cappel, my web designer and creator of the Body Plan website, www.BodyPlanForKids.com.

To Dr. Kevin Stephens and his team of experts at the City of New Orleans Health Department for partnering in this project to bring solid, research-backed programming to address the childhood obesity problem in my city.

And, finally, to Patrick McCausland, general manager of my five GNC franchise stores, who has been instrumental in the follow-through with the Body Plan for Kids' weekly email tips.

My thanks to all of you for helping to bring this book to fruition.

Foreword

While serving as the Health Director for the City of New Orleans, I have had the privilege to work with Mackie Shilstone on several health-related community projects.

Historically, New Orleans has had extremely high rates of childhood obesity. To combat childhood obesity, we have worked with Mackie on several fronts. His Body Plan for Kids program is one key tool to be used to help conquer this problem.

There are many facets to combating obesity, including public policy, parental guidance, community support, school meals and vending policies and, of course, the child. *Mackie Shilstone's Body Plan for Kids* systematically and comprehensively addresses each of these components. Obesity can be quite a complicated and difficult area to address. There are myriads of variables and factors that contribute to this problem. Unfortunately, until now, there were very few tools or resource guides available. *Mackie Shilstone's Body Plan for Kids* is a valuable resource and tool that can be utilized by the entire community.

Our community like many others across America needs a precise, concise, and practical guide to facilitate discussions and actions to reduce the prevalence of childhood obesity. Legislators and policy makers frequently contact me to assist them in developing relevant laws and policies to reduce childhood obesity. There are very few excellent comprehensive resources available. The Body Plan for Kids program fits into this gap.

Churches and other community-based organizations frequently are willing to host or sponsor events and activities designed to promote healthy dietary practices and physical activities. However, in this quest, evidence-based practical guidelines and suggestions have been difficult to obtain. Additionally, many schools have been tasked by parents and concerned citizens to play a greater role in the prevention of childhood obesity. *Mackie Shilstone's Body Plan for Kids* will contribute significantly to these and other organizations as they develop meaningful interventions for our children.

I have had a meaningful and rewarding experience with the Body Plan for Kids program. This book is more than worthy of the highest recommendation. Mr. Shilstone is clearly brilliant at what he does, and has successfully put together a comprehensive nutritional and exercise road map for kids and their caretakers.

The principles in the book are medically sound. Working with children is fun and rewarding; however, it also can present challenges. This book alleviates most and perhaps all the significant challenges one would face. I actually look forward to recommending and supporting the program as outlined in this book. The program can bring about major lifestyle changes for kids that will be lifelong. I highly recommend this book to everyone, particularly to those who are looking to help children get into better shape. This will be one of those life-changing books, which, if its principles are applied, will enable our children not only to get into good shape but also to stay fit for life. Lastly, I want to thank Mr. Shilstone for his superb work in the field and for how much he has helped me, and no doubt countless others.

Kevin U. Stephens, Sr., MD, JD
Director, New Orleans Health Department

INTRODUCTION

What Is the Body Plan for Kids?

For the past thirty years—perhaps even longer—there has been an alarming trend occurring in this country. It is a trend toward childhood obesity that has reached what many experts in the field consider to be an epidemic.

There are many reasons for this epidemic, the most serious of which I will be discussing in this book: primarily, the lack of physical activity among large numbers of young people and the widespread consumption of foods and beverages with little or no nutritional value. Since the road to good health is a lifelong journey that begins at a young age, I have made it my personal crusade to address this rapidly growing problem of obesity at its roots—at the ages when the problems traditionally begin in both boys and girls.

As a professional in the field of performance enhancement and lifestyle management for the past thirty years, I have trained several thousand professional athletes in all major sports, as well as thousands of other individuals. They include four boxing world titleholders, Hall of Famers in baseball and football, All-Star basketball and hockey players, tennis champions and, indeed, entire professional teams. Most of those with whom I have worked are adults, many of whom began developing good exercise and eating habits while they were young. But what about the young people who don't aspire to athletic careers and have developed unhealthy habits at early ages? Those are the ones I am primarily targeting with this book—along with their parents.

The future of our nation depends on the sound physical and mental health of today's generation and the generations to come after them. In order to meet the complex challenges of the world today and tomorrow, our citizens must be in a perpetual state of readiness to confront and overcome those challenges. Sound minds and bodies will be needed to rise up and defend our nation and its way of life against threats to its security, both internal and external. The best insurance against our society "going soft" is to develop the good habits of exercise and healthy eating.

"This is my quest," to quote from the lyrics of the popular song "The Impossible Dream." But my "dream" is not an "impossible" one. It is entirely possible and do-able if the proper steps are taken at an early enough age to set the next generation and those to follow on the proper course. The target audience for this book is primarily those boys and girls in the eight-to-twelve-year-old group—and their parents. While good eating and exercise habits that lead to weight loss and maintaining a healthy weight should begin even sooner and continue for life, I specifically target this age group because studies have shown it to be the ages during which a child's growth and development is at its most active.

Aiming a book at this specific age group requires a different approach than weight-loss books and programs aimed at adults. Kids this age have their own specific nutritional, psychological, and physical needs. As adults, especially those of us whose metabolism has begun to slow down in middle age and unhealthy weight gain has crept up on us, there are constant reminders all around us of the risks of carrying those extra pounds. Children generally aren't confronted with those realities at their age. Even if they're overweight, they—and their parents, very often—may tend to bury their heads in the sand and think that it's just "baby fat" that will come off on its own as they get older. Unfortunately, that frequently isn't the case. Excess pounds put on at an early age may be just the beginning of a pattern that will follow that person throughout his or her life if something isn't done to correct the problem early enough.

My guiding motto throughout this process is that "You fix the apple by fixing the tree": approaching and tackling the problem with a balanced, holistic approach. Parents play a key role in this process, especially, by becoming trainers for their kids as well as for themselves. They must set the example they expect their kids to follow. If they expect their kids to be a healthy weight and keep the unhealthy weight off, they must do likewise. If they expect their kids to exercise, they themselves must exercise. If they expect their kids to eat healthy foods, they must also eat healthy foods.

All these issues and their solutions will be discussed in detail in the chapters that follow. I will recommend physical activities that are simple and non-strenuous, as well as eating guidelines and healthy meal suggestions that will not only help children in the eight-to-twelve-year-old age group maintain a healthy weight but also set them up for a healthy future. Beyond this age group, we will recommend the next tier of intervention.

For assistance in writing this book I assembled a team of experts—a pediatrician, a licensed nutritionist, a child psychiatrist, and other specialists. I also consulted many reputable and highly specialized sources, especially professional journals. My Body Plan for Kids is a hands-on program that has proven to work with parents and their kids, as well as with schools, health professionals, and government public health agencies. It has helped those entities address this problem and come up with workable solutions. It is being promoted through my own facility, The Fitness Principle with Mackie Shilstone, at East Jefferson General Hospital in Metairie, Louisiana. I am confident it can work everywhere else where there is a willingness to apply the principles and steps I lay out.

And, to be sure, some assistance from local, state, and federal government agencies will be needed in this quest, as well. An editorial in the *New York Times* (August 17, 2008), written while the Summer Olympics were being held in Beijing, called upon the public sector to spend more money and pay closer attention to the physical health of our youth instead of subsidizing Olympic athletes—a task best left to the private sector, according to the editorial. "If we are looking to invest in sports, we would be wiser to spend money on daily gym classes and after-school athletic programs," the editorial said. "That would not produce a large crop of Olympians, but it would help combat the growing obesity epidemic among American youngsters and yield health benefits worth more than Olympic gold." To which I wholeheartedly agree.

Maybe there is some glimmer of hope, though, according to a study concluded by the federal Centers for Disease Control and Prevention and published in the *Journal of the American Medical Association*, also in the summer of 2008. That study appeared to show evidence that the percentages of children who are overweight or obese may be leveling off and holding steady for the first time since 1980. Schools serving healthier meals and upgrading physical education programs was believed to be one of the causative factors in this development. However, until those numbers start going down significantly, we will still have a long way to go in solving this problem.

Lastly, I need to emphasize that my Body Plan for Kids is not a specific diet or exercise program. There are plenty of those out there in the marketplace today, most of which appear to work for large numbers of people. My aim is to put the problem out there for all to see, to closely examine its causes and effects, and then offer general guidelines and suggestions as to how the problem can be corrected. This is the best service that I can offer. I hope I am successful in getting this word out and I will be relying heavily on you for reader feedback to let me know if my program is working for you and your kids. You can write to me in care of the publisher or to me directly at my website www.BodyPlanForKids.com. I welcome your comments, suggestions, and words of encouragement, and I thank you for taking the time to read this book.

PART ONE

Childhood Obesity: What Parents Need to Know

CHAPTER 1

Common Causes and Consequences of Childhood Obesity

Finding Solutions to a National Epidemic

Childhood obesity is a "national epidemic." These are not just my words, but the words of many health professionals, organizations, and medical practitioners. It is an epidemic that has already started to have serious consequences, and may have even more serious consequences in the future if something isn't done about it *now*. If this trend isn't reversed, a sizable percentage of the next generation to guide the destiny of the United States may experience serious health-related issues that will negatively impact their longevity.

Today, more than one in three children and adolescents in the United States is considered overweight or obese, according to a number of studies. This translates roughly into about 25 million children. The Atlanta-based Centers for Disease Control and Prevention now estimate that approximately 19 percent of children (ages six to eleven) and 17 percent of adolescents (ages twelve to nineteen) are considered overweight or obese. These numbers have nearly tripled among children and quadrupled among adolescents during the last twenty-five years. And the figures for African-American and Hispanic children show nearly double the rates of overweight and obesity. These are significant numbers, and they could grow even larger at the present rate.

The worst part about all this is the long-term health repercussions. Overweight and obese children can grow into overweight and obese adults if their eating and exercise habits don't change. Obesity can lead to increased risks for coronary heart disease, hypertension (high blood pressure), type 2 diabetes, asthma, sleep disorders, elevated levels of harmful LDL cholesterol, and other serious medical problems. Metabolism, normally at high levels in youngsters, can be slowed down by these risk factors, and serious imbalances in the endocrine (hormonal) system can also result. Shorter life expectancy may be the final result of any one or combination of these obesity-related disorders.

WHY KIDS ARE MORE OBESE TODAY

There are many reasons why kids are more obese today than those of previous generations, not the least of which may be attributable to the relative affluence we now enjoy. Many of today's kids are engaged in sedentary pursuits made possible by a level of technology unthinkable as recently as twenty-five to thirty years ago. Computer, video, and other virtual games, the ready availability of feature films and games on DVD, plus high-tech advancements in music-listening technology, have come down into the range of affordability for parents and even for the kids themselves. These passive pursuits have produced a downside of reduced physical activity for the kids, often with the explicit or implicit consent of the parents.

During the time of this generation's parents' parents and grandparents, these luxuries did not exist. Physical activity was more the rule than the exception. Sports were encouraged, with fathers and even grandfathers teaching their sons and grandsons baseball, football, basketball, tennis, swimming, or other games and activities that gave the kids a healthy workout. Girls were steered into certain sports like volleyball, basketball (if they were tall), gymnastics, and swimming, or other physical activities like dance, jump rope, or cheerleading. Families went camping, hiking, or biking together.

Television, in the 1950s and '60s, was a relatively new development and a luxury that families were only gradually able to afford. The early shows that families watched together emphasized healthy values that often included physical activity. Parents on many of these shows would go out to watch their sons play baseball or football, and the kids watching these shows often aspired to be athletic themselves because of what they were seeing.

The schools at that time were doing their part, as well. For many of us during that generation, physical education was *mandatory*. Not just for one or two years, but for the entire four years of high school. It was as much a part of the academic curriculum as math, science, and social studies. Even those children who engaged in no other physical activities outside of school were assured of at least two or three hours of some type of exercise a week. Five to ten minutes of warm-up calisthenics often preceded forty to fifty minutes of whatever sport or activity was in the curriculum for that quarter or semester.

Today, phys ed or "gym" has virtually disappeared from many of our nation's primary and secondary schools. In a number of states and individual school districts, it is no longer mandatory, and in some schools is not even an option. To their credit, most schools still have extracurricular programs in various sports, but only those students who go out for those sports get the benefit of physical activity. (See Appendix B for the physical education requirements for your state.)

Other fairly recent developments have also contributed to the alarming rise in child obesity rates. Fast food outlets offering consumables that are both low in price and low in nutritional content have exploded all over the American landscape since the 1960s, especially in suburban areas close to major highway interchanges. Kids on their lunch breaks or after school often congregate in these fast food outlets, consuming food and soft drinks that are high in sugar, carbohydrates, and fat. Many parents, themselves, frequently take their children to these fast food places, thus setting an example the kids can find justification to emulate.

In years past, before fast foods became as widespread as they are now, families sat down to healthy, home-cooked meals together. Food items did not have all the additives and artificial ingredients they do now. Livestock and other live animals processed for food were not injected with chemicals designed to make their meat more visually appealing. Juices advertised as such were just that, not flavored water with little or no actual fruit content. Most sweetened products contained real, organic sugar, not the high-fructose corn syrup and other artificial sweeteners so widely used today. Many products sold as "health foods" today—usually at higher prices than conventional food items—were standard fare thirty or forty years ago. The "building blocks" of good nutrition were widely pub-licized and many parents did their best to abide by them in preparing meals for themselves and their offspring.

For many years, a vast number of school lunch programs served meals that focused more on cost than nutritional value. In order to save money, school districts often order food that is cheap to prepare and serve. Late-ly, many school districts have begun offering healthy alternatives to the less nutritional fare they've served in the past, but if the kids aren't encouraged to eat healthy they may continue consuming the "junk food" they've always eaten. Vitamins and supplements that might help kids make up for the nutrients they're not getting from food sources are usually not on their agenda. The parents, themselves, make up the largest share of the market for supplements, and it is usually the parents who have to acquire the sup-plements for the kids and make sure they take them.

People of earlier generations ate not only more whole, nutrient-dense foods, but also smaller quantities of it. Twenty years ago, for example, the portion size of a bagel was 3 inches; a soda, 6.5 ounces; and a cheeseburger was simply a cheeseburger. Today, the portion size of a bagel is 6 inches; a soda, 20 ounces; and a cheeseburger has become a double cheeseburger.

Childhood obesity has become so widespread today that many par-ents don't even realize that their children are obese. A poll taken by *Con-sumer Reports* in July 2007, involving over 3,000 parents of overweight or obese children between the ages of five and seventeen, showed that close to half of them didn't consider their children to be overweight. Those conducting the study think it might be because there are so many other overweight children among their kids' peers. To these parents, their kids look fairly normal and healthy.

In many of these borderline cases, it's difficult to fault the parents. They may have been raised to "eat hearty" by parents who grew up dur-ing the Great Depression when food and the money to buy it with were scarce. It's perfectly natural for parents to want the best for their kids and to try to make their kids' lives easier and better than they might have had it. Today, many parents have the means to better provide for their chil-dren, and they do so by giving them more than they might have gotten when they were their kids' ages.

The constant bombardment of advertisements on TV and in other media consciously and relentlessly feed into this sentiment. It's as if they're saying, "If you love your kids, you will buy them this." Love is equated with money and material possessions. These ad techniques must be working because they've been with us for many years. Eager to please their children and see the happy smiles on their faces at birthdays or on Christmas morning, parents will buy them motorized three-wheeler dirt bikes instead of manually operated bicycles that give the kids needed physical exercise. They'll buy them DVDs and iPods instead of basketball hoops or punching bags or sets of weights. The list goes on and on.

Our present-day affluence has made it possible for our kids to have their own TV sets, personal computers, sound equipment, calculators, and other devices that encourage passive pursuits. Our kids' generation is growing up with computers like our generation grew up with typewriters, and many of today's classrooms have their own computers or laptop hookups. The upside of this is the marvelous advancement in learning technology; facts and information are readily accessible with the click of a mouse button. No more long hours spent in the library poring through hundreds of pages from books to gather information for term papers. The downside of this computer technology is that too many kids are spending *too much* time at it and not enough time doing things that are beneficial to their physical health.

What I have witnessed, particularly over the past ten years while my own two sons were growing up, is that fewer and fewer kids play outside or take part in outdoor activities that challenge them physically. It dismays me to see so few of these kids playing touch football or basketball, or engaging in activities that involve running. Too many of these kids are becoming proficient in exercises involving the hands but overall are becoming movement inefficient in exercises for the whole body. In the process, they may be slowing down their metabolic rate by assuming seated positions for long periods of time. Consequently, the more weight they gain, the more they may be contributing to lower back pain.

In addition to penalizing themselves physically, kids who are heavily involved in sedentary activities are also depriving themselves of opportunities to learn the importance of teamwork and cooperation with their peers. Team sports teach these skills and allow kids to experience the thrill of working toward the common goal of winning. Computer games are usually one against one. A few sports like boxing and tennis match one individual's skills against another, but most sports require the joint effort only a team pulling together can achieve.

Many computer games also give kids an unrealistic dose of unreality. You can be killed in a war game yet get up and start fighting again. Of course, as we all know, it isn't like that in the real world. The sedentary lifestyle many of today's kids are living can become a symptom of a much larger problem—a concentration of metabolic disorders that become silent killers at earlier ages than in years' past. With these conditions, you don't get shot down and get back up again.

THE TOLL ON OUR CHILDREN'S HEALTH

This inattention to caloric intake, nutritious foods, and physical activity has begun to take its toll in only a single generation. According to James S. Marks, MD, MPH, senior vice president and director of the Robert Wood Johnson Foundation's health group, "If we don't deal with the problem, this could be the first generation that will live sicker and die younger than its parents." The foundation recently announced a massive effort to reduce the childhood obesity epidemic by 2015. Between now and then, it plans to spend $500 million on public-health initiatives focusing on kids and families in underserved communities.

A child who is overweight or obese is at risk of developing, as soon as young adulthood:

- High blood pressure: This condition is damaging to blood vessel walls, especially in the heart, and is one of the most important risk factors for heart attacks and strokes. In a recent study undertaken by the Tulane University School of Medicine in New Orleans, researchers documented a significant upward trend over the past sixteen years in blood pressure levels of children and teens between the ages of eight and eighteen. The study team concluded that this trend may be largely attributed to the increase in the number of overweight and obese children over the same time period.

- High cholesterol: Studies have shown that fatty plaque buildup begins in childhood and progresses slowly into adulthood. This disease process is called atherosclerosis and is caused by high levels of "bad" LDL (low-density lipoprotein) cholesterol and low levels of "good" HDL (high-density lipoprotein) cholesterol. In time, atherosclerosis leads to heart disease, which is the single biggest cause of death in the United States. A study presented at the American Heart Association Conference in New Orleans in November 2008 found that the thickness of artery walls in children who are obese or have high cholesterol resembled the thickness of artery walls of an average forty-five-year-old. Findings from another study presented at the conference found that children who were obese had greater enlargement of their hearts.

- Insulin resistance/type 2 diabetes: The full impact of the childhood obesity epidemic has yet to be seen, because it can take up to ten years or longer for obese individuals to develop type 2 diabetes. However, children who are obese today are more likely to develop type 2 diabetes as young adults. The longer a person has diabetes, the more likely he or she is to develop serious complications such as kidney failure and blindness. That means that young adults with type 2 diabetes are much more likely to develop such complications during their lifetime than older people with the disease. (More on insulin resistance/type 2 diabetes in Chapter 3.)

- Asthma: Studies show that overweight children are more likely to be asthmatic than healthy weight children. Obesity can impact lung function in a variety of ways. One common argument is that obese children are less likely to exercise, which may have some effect on the condition. Obesity is also thought to constrict airways.

- Sleep disorders: Obesity can increase children's risk for developing obstructive sleep apnea (OSA), a sleep-related breathing disorder that causes your body to stop breathing during sleep. The lungs in an overweight or obese person are forced to work harder during sleep than they are in a person of low or normal weight. OSA, which can disturb your sleep numerous times on any given night, can result in daytime sleepiness.

- Kidney disease: (Related to type-2 diabetes: see above.)

- Long-term weight problems: The number of fat cells, or adipocytes, in the body is set during childhood. Once the fat cell is there it's there forever. You don't lose fat cells; you lose fat from fat cells. Less than 10 percent of children with normal weight go on to develop adult obesity, whereas an estimated 80 percent of obese children will become and remain overweight as adults, if no intervention is made in time.

- Shortened lifespan: A 2005 study that was co-authored by David Ludwig, MD, PhD, associate professor of pediatrics at Harvard University, predicted that obesity could shorten the average child's lifespan by two to five years.

Other studies, both here and abroad, have reached roughly the same conclusions about childhood obesity and its causes and effects. Although specific findings may vary and percentages may differ from one study to the next, the message is nonetheless clear: children must be taught lifelong fitness and healthy eating habits at home and their parents must play a proactive role in this process.

WHAT PARENTS CAN DO

Over the years, our culture has misguidedly defined health by body size and weight. Many of our well-intentioned Old World grandparents, themselves often coming from impoverished homes where food of any type was scarce, identified overweight children as being healthy. Indeed, in the nineteenth and early twentieth centuries—and at various other times in the history of the Western world—being fat was considered both fashionable and a sign of wealth and prosperity. And, yes, even a sign of good health! Even today, despite the vast body of medical evidence to the contrary, many parents and grandparents consider overweight babies to be healthy ones. "Baby fat" is just something "they will grow out of as they get older," they confidently assume. And, in so assuming, they may conveniently excuse themselves from dealing with a very real problem they think will automatically solve itself.

Well, it just doesn't automatically work that way. Sometimes kids actually do lose their baby fat as they get older, but many don't. Not without help, anyway. This is where parents have to step in and become more proactive.

What can parents do to help their offspring become leaner and fitter? The answer is, many things, starting with their own habits and lifestyles. Parents must make it a point to educate themselves on the values of healthy eating and exercise and discontinue bad habits—for their children as well as for themselves. If they smoke or consume alcohol to excess, they must quit. If they eat unhealthy foods or consume non-nutritious soft drinks, they need to switch to healthier consumables with higher levels of essential nutrients. If they sit for long periods watching TV or working on the computer, they need to get up and start doing some form of physical exercise. Only by setting an example themselves can parents become the role models they want their kids to follow. If they don't, some researchers warn, in ten to twenty years an entire generation of young adults may suffer from major health problems that were formerly associated with middle or advanced age.

Parents must learn to recognize what is and what isn't a healthy weight or body mass index (the most widely used diagnostic tool to identify weight problems) for their kids. But it isn't just the parents who need to learn these facts. Unfortunately, many healthcare providers aren't up to speed on this, either. In the *Consumer Reports* study cited earlier, only 36 percent of the surveyed parents with overweight kids said their doctors suggested that the child lose weight. The other 64 percent say the doctor didn't mention it.

Thus, it would appear that there is a serious disconnect between those who should know the facts about childhood obesity and the facts themselves. In cases like these, it would be difficult to fault the media. There is a plethora of valuable information out there. Every week there are dozens of articles on childhood health published in widely read media or on frequently viewed websites. There are hundreds more if you count technical and trade journals. The information and facts are there—they're just not being read and put into practice frequently enough by those who should be reading and practicing them. Granted, reading about health issues is not as entertaining or titillating as reading about celebrities, but, in terms of how our children are affected, this is far more important. For ourselves as well as for them.

Once parents have educated themselves on what they need to do to help make their kids (and themselves) healthier and to start practicing good eating and exercising habits, they need to devise programs for their kids to follow. Some of these programs could and should involve activities—both physical and nutritional—that parents and kids can do together. For the programs that cannot be done together, parents need to closely monitor their kids' food and beverage intake levels, as well as their activities. TV viewing and computer usage can be regulated to an essential minimum and balanced against quality periods of physical activity. Parents should encourage their kids to learn as much as they can about nutrition, and the kids should aid their parents in planning healthy, balanced meals. Visits to fast food outlets need to be regulated and kept to a manageable minimum.

In the chapters to come, I will discuss many aspects of the problem of childhood overweight and obesity and what can be done about them. For parents who want to learn even more about these problems, I refer you to the Resources section in the back of this book.

CHAPTER 1 SUMMARY

- Childhood obesity is a national epidemic with more than one in three children considered to be overweight.

- Obesity can lead to increased risks for coronary heart disease, hypertension, type 2 diabetes, asthma, sleep disorders, elevated levels of harmful cholesterol, and other serious health issues.

- Lifestyles have changed. Children today are less physically active than in the past and are eating foods that are low in nutrition and high in sugar, fats, and carbohydrates.

- It is important that parents get involved and educate themselves on proper nutrition and exercise so that they can be a good role model for their children.

CHAPTER 2

Genetics and Metabolic Imbalances

Identifying Other Factors That Cause Childhood Obesity

The trend toward childhood obesity should be of particular concern to the parents of children who fit into this category, yet many parents are unsure what causes their kids to be obese or borderline overweight, and what they can do about it. Is it simple overeating? Is it hereditary, something in the family's genes? Is it a result of unhealthy lifestyle choices? Or is it a combination of all or some of these physical and environmental factors? The problem, most experts will insist, is a combination of the above factors.

While the most common causes of overweight and obesity are poor diet and/or eating habits and a lack of exercise, there are factors that may be more difficult to control such as your child's genetic makeup or their individual body chemistry that might be causing his or her weight problem.

THE GENETIC CONNECTION

There is almost no dispute that obesity may be in the genes that are transmitted from one generation to the next. In many cases, just a casual observation of these families will appear to confirm that, and detailed studies also appear to back up the genetic issues, as well.

In a 2001 joint study between Louisiana State University and the University of Oulu in Finland, sponsored by the Nestlé Corporation, it was stated that "Most (family) studies support the notion that there is

17

a significant genetic component in the development of obesity . . .
Undoubtedly, the development of obesity results from the combined
effects of predisposing genes, behavioral factors, and their interactions."
The study also suggests that the problem of obesity in a child is com-
pounded when both parents are overweight. In such cases, the risks of the
child developing into an overweight adult may be as much as doubled.

Even more recently, scientists and researchers in Great Britain isolated what is believed to be the "obesity gene," the genetic component
that predisposes certain individuals toward obesity. In an April 12, 2007
article in *Science*, the journal of the American Association for the Advancement of Science, a U.K. research team, led by Dr. Andrew Hattersley of
Peninsula Medical School in Exeter, reported the discovery of a gene
variant that occurs in over half of people of European descent, which
they think helps to regulate the amount of fat in the body.

The scientists discovered the gene, known as FTO, in a study of 2,000
diabetics when they were doing a search for susceptibility to type 2 diabetes. They found there was a strong link between the FTO variant and
body mass index (BMI). They conducted another study on thirteen
groups of 38,759 Britons, Finns, and Italians, aged seven and older, and
found a similar link between the FTO variant and increased body weight.
Those who were found to have this gene had a 70 percent higher risk of
being obese and were on average 6.5 pounds heavier than those who
didn't have it.

However, just because someone carries this gene variant doesn't
mean they are predestined to be overweight and stay that way. A study
conducted a year later by a research team from the University of Maryland yielded some optimistic findings. Headed by Soren Snitker, MD,
PhD, and his postdoctoral fellow, Evadnie Rampersaud, MSPH, PhD,
who is now of the University of Miami, the team studied 704 Amish men
and women who carried the FTO gene. The researchers found that the
most physically active men and women were able to stay within a normal
BMI range despite their genetic predisposition, while those who were
relatively inactive were overweight. The study results were published in
the *Archives of Internal Medicine* in September 2008.

Genetics is a complicated and controversial field that we have only recently begun to understand. It has been known since earliest times that physical characteristics such as hair, eye, and skin color are frequently passed on from one generation to the next. Intelligence, creativity, athletic abilities, and other physical and mental attributes or deficiencies can be passed on as well. Casual observation will confirm this. So do studies, such as the study conducted at the Free University of Amsterdam, the Netherlands, that make a strong case for the passing down of athletic ability from one generation to the next.

What still remains to be discovered, is exactly *how* these traits are passed on. Studies of chromosomes involved in genetics have helped unlock some of these mysteries, but much more study needs to be done. And, the more that is learned about genetics, the greater the fears voiced by certain segments of the population. Genetic engineering (human cloning) is a sensitive subject, which conjures up "Brave New World" images of a conformist, amorphous society that can easily be controlled if genetically programmed a certain way. There are also those for whom human cloning violates their religious beliefs, and these individuals and groups make up a large segment of the population.

Perhaps, though, in a positive way, genetic engineering may eventually be able to alter a predisposition to obesity in those with obese parents and/or grandparents. However, we can't wait for that day to come. Despite obesity being a family trait, there is no reason to throw one's hands in the air and presume that nothing can be done about it. Obesity *can* be controlled and reduced, even if it "runs in the family." It can be managed through proper dietary habits and physical exercise, as I will expound on later in this book. My thirty-plus years of experience in the performance enhancement field have produced many excellent examples of this.

METABOLIC IMBALANCES

Our bodies get the energy they need from food through metabolism, the chemical reactions in the body's cells that convert the fuel from food into the energy needed to do everything from moving to thinking. Several hormones of the endocrine system are involved in controlling the rate of metabolism. A metabolic disorder is any disease that is caused by an abnormal chemical reaction in the body's cells. Most disorders of metabolism involve either abnormal levels of enzymes or hormones, or problems with the functioning of those enzymes or hormones, which can lead to serious problems.

Two disorders of the endocrine system may be factors in a predisposition toward obesity: hypothyroidism and insulin resistance (diabetes).

Hypothyroidism

Imbalances in thyroid hormone can interfere with the body's metabolic processes and decrease the body's ability to function efficiently. It has been known for a very long time that there is a complex relationship between thyroid disease, body weight, and metabolism. Thyroid hormones regulate metabolism in both animals and humans. People with an underactive thyroid (hypothyroidism) tend to have a very low basal metabolic rate. This, if not controlled, may lead to weight gain in children as well as adults. An individual's metabolic rate will very often determine their body weight and body mass index. The slower one's metabolism is, the longer excess fat remains in the body, and the more likely they are to be overweight or obese.

In addition to possible weight gain, other common symptoms of hypothyroidism may include:

• Fatigue

• Depression

• Muscle weakness

• Poor appetite

• Dry skin

• Cold intolerance

• Dry or brittle hair

• Hair loss

- Constipation

- Muscle cramps

- Delayed puberty

- Poor school performance (dropping grades, etc.)

It is estimated that one child in every 4,000 is born with hypothyroidism and within a few weeks or months about 10 percent of them will lose the condition. However, it remains a serious risk for many young children and older adolescents. A comprehensive medical examination and thyroid function tests may help determine if indeed your child has a thyroid imbalance and, if so, what you might need to counterbalance it. A number of prescription drugs can be taken that won't negatively impact your child's ability to exercise and eat the right foods.

Insulin Resistance

Insulin resistance is another factor that may lead to obesity in kids. Insulin is the hormone that enables cells in the body to absorb glucose (blood sugar) and nutrients from digested foods. It is produced in the pancreas and, during puberty, the pancreas produces more insulin than usual, which helps account for children's growth spurts at that age. High and low insulin levels are frequently associated with the different types of diabetes. Insulin resistance is defined as "the inability of circulating insulin to exert a normal physiological effect at a target tissue, classically described as impaired insulin-stimulated skeletal muscle glucose uptake." In layman's terms, this simply means that those who are defined as "insulin resistant" have difficulty breaking down food in their bodies, which may lead to that food being stored as fat, which then leads to unhealthy weight gain.

Insulin sensitivity is the opposite of insulin resistance. It doesn't generally cause weight gain but it is important to mention here nonetheless. The more insulin sensitive an individual is, generally speaking, the better their digestive systems' enzymes break down food into its essential components—amino acids from proteins, fatty acids from fats, and simple sugars (glucose) from carbohydrates. These compounds are used as energy sources by the body when needed. They are absorbed into the blood, which transports them to the cells. After they enter the cells, other enzymes act to speed up or regulate the chemical reactions involved with metabolizing these compounds. During these processes, the energy from these compounds can be released for use by the body or stored in body tissues, especially the liver, muscles, and body fat. So, the more insulin sensitive an individual is, the less prone to unhealthy weight gain they may be.

There are a number of disorders associated with the body's ability or inability to process insulin, the most common and best known of which are the two forms of diabetes (diabetes mellitus): type 1 and type 2.

Type 1 diabetes occurs when the pancreas produces and secretes little or no insulin. Type 1 is sometimes referred to as "juvenile diabetes" because it primarily affects kids, although it can affect adults as well. Symptoms of this disease may include excessive thirst and urination, hunger, and weight loss. Over the long term, the disease can cause kidney problems, pain due to nerve damage, blindness, and heart and blood vessel disease. Kids and teens with type 1 diabetes need to receive regular injections of insulin and control blood sugar levels to reduce the risk of developing problems from diabetes. Type 1 diabetes is the less common of the two types, comprising only 5 to 10 percent of all diabetes cases. It is believed to stem almost entirely from genetic factors, but type 1 diabetes is not normally associated with weight gain. The main purpose for mentioning it here is to differentiate it from the more common type 2 diabetes.

Type 2 diabetes occurs when the body can no longer respond normally to insulin. The symptoms of this disorder are similar to those of type 1 diabetes, except that many children and teens who develop type 2 diabetes are overweight, and this is thought to play a role in their decreased responsiveness to insulin. Some kids and teens can be treated successfully with dietary changes, exercise, and oral medication, but insulin injections are necessary in other cases. Controlling blood sugar levels reduces the risk of developing the same kinds of long-term health problems that occur with type 1 diabetes.

Type 2 diabetes, unfortunately, is most often a lifetime condition. Those who have it must either endure injections for the rest of their lives or take prescription medicines similar to insulin but with potentially undesirable side effects. Medical science has not yet developed an insulin pill or capsule that can be taken orally and have the same effect as an injection. Insulin is absorbed very rapidly once it enters the body and, if taken orally, it would break down in the digestive process before it reached its intended target. However, medical scientists are determined to develop an effective insulin pill and they are confident that it's just a matter of time before they do. In the meantime, insulin pumps, patches, and sprays are non-intrusive ways of getting insulin into the bloodstream, but they are more costly and possibly less effective than the more commonly used injection methods.

A comprehensive medical examination that can diagnose diabetes, or glycemic disorders that can lead to diabetes, is strongly recommended for all children at an early age. The sooner diabetes or other forms of insulin resistance are diagnosed, the more effectively they can be treated. Robert Gensure, MD, head of the Department of Pediatric Endocrinology at the Ochsner Clinic Foundation in New Orleans, confirms that overweight children are at a higher risk of developing diabetes in the future if they don't get their weight under control while they're still young. "That's what we're trying to do: pick them up at that stage and keep them from getting diabetes," Dr. Gensure noted. "We have measures to try to prevent this and weight control reduces that risk about 70 to 75 percent."

Nonetheless, having diabetes or insulin resistance does not mean that a person can't lose weight. With proper diet and regular exercise that takes the condition into account, unnecessary weight gain can be minimized, if not prevented totally. Any weight loss program involving diabetics or others who are insulin resistant should be done under a doctor's close supervision.

WHAT PARENTS CAN DO

Dealing with a weight problem that is precipitated by your child's genetic makeup or individual body chemistry may be more difficult to control than just controlling their TV viewing time or the foods they eat. Exercise and proper nutrition can usually help kids with these conditions, but they may also need prescription medicines and intense supervision by those in the medical profession. Nevertheless, there are many things parents can do to help their children lead healthier, happier lives. Below I offer some strategies and guidelines parents can follow that empower their children to take concrete steps to developing healthier habits, all of which I will discuss in depth in later chapters.

- Get a pediatric evaluation of your child to make sure that his or her obesity does not have a physical cause.

- Learn to be positive. Instead of nagging children and making them feel self-conscious about their weight, parents can focus on the positive benefits of good nutrition and increased activity, such as feeling healthier, happier, and stronger.

- Become a better consumer. It is important for parents to educate their children about the unrealistic and harmful effects of media images of perfection, and instead stress the value of developing positive inner qualities. They can also help their kids to become more aware of how television, magazine, and online ads can make unhealthy foods seem appealing.

- Make eating healthfully a family affair. Instead of singling out the overweight child, parents can make better nutritional choices for the entire family. Also, parents can get the whole family involved in more outings that involve physical activity.

- Avoid using food as either a reward or a punishment.

- Make mealtimes a pleasant family affair, a time of togetherness uninterrupted by phone calls and TV programs.

- Get kids involved in creating interesting and healthier food choices and teach them how to read and interpret ingredient data and nutritional information on package labels. Chapter 6 on Recipes Kids Love will make this job easier for parents.

CHAPTER 2 SUMMARY

- Childhood obesity has become so widespread that many parents do not even realize that their child is obese.

- The most common causes of childhood overweight and obesity are poor diet and lack of exercise, but there may be other factors that may be more difficult to control.

- Hormonal imbalances, such as thyroid problems, can interfere with the body's metabolic processes and decrease its ability to function efficiently possibly causing weight gain.

- Insulin sensitivity/resistance is a factor that may lead to obesity in kids due to the difficulty of breaking down food increasing the possibility of fat production.

- Nonetheless, weight loss is still attainable with proper nutrition, physical activity and the adaptation of a more positive lifestyle.

PART TWO

Physical and Mental Evaluations

CHAPTER 3

How Does Your Kid Measure Up?

Evaluating Your Child's Weight and Fat Patterns

The problem of childhood obesity is growing (literally!) by the day. Some researchers predict that nearly half the children in North American will be overweight by 2010, and data indicates that 80 percent of these children will likely be overweight adults, placing them at a higher risk of developing health problems like high cholesterol, hypertension, and type 2 diabetes.

Much, if not most, of the responsibility for getting a handle on this problem lies with the parents. The first step to solving a problem is identifying it. But how does a parent evaluate whether their child is just a bit overweight, significantly overweight, or medically obese? What are some of the danger signs that your child might be developing a weight problem and, if so, what is causing it?

Before I answer the second question, let me address the first one. We must start out by defining what is "overweight" and what is "obese." Though they may appear to be synonyms and interchangeable in a general sense, medically they don't mean the same thing. Instead they define different degrees of being above an acceptable weight level: different percentiles of the population within specific age groups.

OVERWEIGHT AND OBESITY DEFINED

In 2007, the American Medical Association (AMA) Expert Committee on

29

the Assessment, Prevention, and Treatment of Child and Adolescent Overweight and Obesity drafted a landmark report with a number of significant recommendations for health-care providers to apply in their practices. The committee, which had been convened by the AMA in collaboration with the Department of Health and Human Services' Health Resources and Services Administration (HRSA) and the Centers for Disease Control and Prevention (CDC), was made up of representatives from fifteen health professional organizations involved in medicine, nutrition, mental health, epidemiology, and psychology. Their goal was to identify new treatment and prevention options to address the growing problem of overweight and obese children. In this important report, the committee defined "overweight" and "obese" and differentiated between the two terms.

The report, which will be discussed further in later chapters and is published in full in Appendix A, states that "Individuals from the ages of two to eighteen years, with a body mass index (BMI) equal to or greater than the 95th percentile for age and sex, or a BMI exceeding 30 (whichever is smaller), should be considered obese. Individuals with a BMI equal to or greater than the 85th percentile, but less than the 95th percentile for age and sex, should be considered overweight." The report added that the term "overweight" replaces "at risk for overweight." What this translates to is that, without lowering the percentile or range, individuals who were once considered to be "at risk" for being overweight are now considered to be overweight. The definition of "overweight" has changed, according to the report.

What does this mean and what do these percentiles indicate? Let us first define what is meant by body mass index.

BMI is a statistical measurement which compares a person's weight and height. Though it does not actually measure the percentage of body fat, it is a useful tool to estimate a healthy body weight based on how tall a person is. Due to its ease of measurement and calculation, the BMI is the most widely used diagnostic tool to identify obesity problems within a population. Although it is not considered appropriate to use as a final indication for diagnosing children, it can be used to identify possible weight problems.

DETERMINING YOUR CHILD'S WEIGHT

The first step to determining whether your child's weight is a health concern is to get accurate measurements of their height and weight. If they have been to a doctor recently, you can get the latest measurements from him or her. If you do this at home, here's how to measure *height* accurately to calculate BMI-for-age:

STEP 1. Get accurate height and weight measurements

1. Remove the child's shoes, bulky clothing, and hair ornaments, and unbraid hair that interferes with the measurement.

2. Take the height measurement on flooring that is not carpeted and against a flat surface such as a wall with no molding.

3. Have the child stand with feet flat, together, and against the wall. Make sure legs are straight, arms are at sides, and shoulders are level.

4. Make sure the child is looking straight ahead and that the line of sight is parallel with the floor.

5. Take the measurement while the child stands with head, shoulders, buttocks, and heels touching the flat surface (wall). Depending on the overall body shape of the child, all points may not touch the wall.

6. Use a flat headpiece such as a ruler or flat sheet of cardboard to form a right angle with the wall and lower the headpiece until it firmly touches the crown of the head.

7. Make sure the measurer's eyes are at the same level as the headpiece.

8. Lightly mark where the bottom of the headpiece meets the wall. Then, use a metal tape to measure from the base of the floor to the marked measurement on the wall to get the height measurement.

9. Accurately record the height to the nearest $1/8$ inch or 0.1 centimeter.

To measure *weight* accurately at home to calculate BMI-for-age:

1. Use a digital scale. Avoid using spring-loaded bathroom scales. Place the scale on firm flooring (such as tile or wood) rather than carpet.

2. Have the child remove shoes and heavy clothing, such as sweaters.

3. Have the child stand with both feet in the center of the scale.

4. Record the weight to the nearest decimal fraction (for example, 55.5 pounds or 25.1 kilograms).

STEP 2. Determine your child's body mass index

The next step is determining your child's BMI. You'll need the height and weight measurements from Step 1.

You can calculate your child's BMI by dividing their weight, in pounds, by the square of their height, in inches, then multiplying by 703. But, if you're not a math major and don't want to go to that trouble, log on to my website at www.BodyPlanForKids.com/article.php?story=bmi calc-children. The computer will automatically calculate the BMI for you.

Once you know your child's BMI, double check it against Table 3.1 on the opposite page. To read the chart: find your child's height in inches, along the left side, and their weight in pounds, across that row. Find where the two numbers intersect, then scroll up to the top of the column. The number in the shaded area is your child's BMI. Use this number to find the category directly above it that defines your child's weight.

To see how your child measures up with other children his or her age, consult the tables on the following pages. These charts were developed by the National Center for Health Statistics, in collaboration with the National Center for Chronic Disease Prevention and Health Promotion, and are considered the industry standard for such measurements.

To read the BMI-for-age percentiles charts for boys (Table 3.2) or girls (Table 3.3), find your child's BMI along the left or right side. Follow the straight line to where it intersects with your child's age, listed across the bottom. The numbers within the curved lines in the column between ages eighteen and nineteen are the BMI percentiles they fall into.

TABLE 3.1. BODY MASS INDEX

To calculate your Body Mass Index (BMI), divide your weight (in pounds) by the square of your height (in inches). Then multiply by 703.

BMI = (weight in pounds) / (height in inches x height in inches) x 703

BMI	Category	BMI	Category
18.5 or less	Underweight	30.0–34.9	Obese
18.5–24.9	Normal	35.0–39.9	Obese
25.0–29.9	Overweight	40 or greater	Extremely Obese

BMI (KG/M²)	19	20	21	22	23	24	25	26	27	28	29	30	35	40
HEIGHT (IN.)						WEIGHT (LB.)								
58	91	96	100	105	110	115	119	124	129	134	138	143	167	191
59	94	99	104	109	114	119	124	128	133	138	143	148	173	198
60	97	102	107	112	118	123	128	133	138	143	148	153	179	204
61	100	106	111	116	122	127	132	137	143	148	153	158	185	211
62	104	109	115	120	126	131	136	142	147	153	158	164	191	218
63	107	113	118	124	130	135	141	146	152	158	163	169	197	225
64	110	116	122	128	134	140	145	151	157	163	169	174	204	232
65	114	120	126	132	138	144	150	156	162	168	174	180	210	240
66	118	124	130	136	142	148	155	161	167	173	179	186	216	247
67	121	127	134	140	146	153	159	166	172	178	185	191	223	255
68	125	131	138	144	151	158	164	171	177	184	190	197	230	262
69	128	135	142	149	155	162	169	176	182	189	196	203	236	270
70	132	139	146	153	160	167	174	181	188	195	202	207	243	278
71	136	143	150	157	165	172	179	186	193	200	208	215	250	286
72	140	147	154	162	169	177	184	191	199	206	213	221	258	294
73	144	151	159	166	174	182	189	197	204	212	219	227	265	302
74	148	155	163	171	179	186	194	202	210	218	225	233	272	311
75	152	160	168	176	184	192	200	208	216	224	232	240	279	319
76	156	164	172	180	189	197	205	213	221	230	238	246	287	328

TABLE 3.2. BMI INDEX-FOR-AGE PERCENTILES FOR BOYS (AGES 2 TO 20)

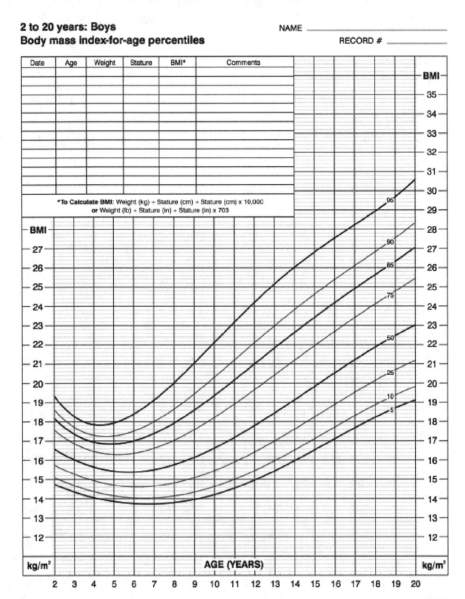

2 to 20 years: Boys
Body mass index-for-age percentiles

NAME _____

RECORD # _____

*To Calculate BMI: Weight (kg) ÷ Stature (cm) ÷ Stature (cm) x 10,000
or Weight (lb) ÷ Stature (in) ÷ Stature (in) x 703

AGE (YEARS)

Published May 30, 2000 (modified 10/16/00).
SOURCE: Developed by the National Center for Health Statistics in collaboration with
the National Center for Chronic Disease Prevention and Health Promotion (2000).
http://www.cdc.gov/growthcharts

SAFER · HEALTHIER · PEOPLE

TABLE 3.3. BMI INDEX-FOR-AGE PERCENTILES FOR GIRLS (AGES 2 TO 20)

2 to 20 years: Girls
Body mass index-for-age percentiles

NAME _____

RECORD # _____

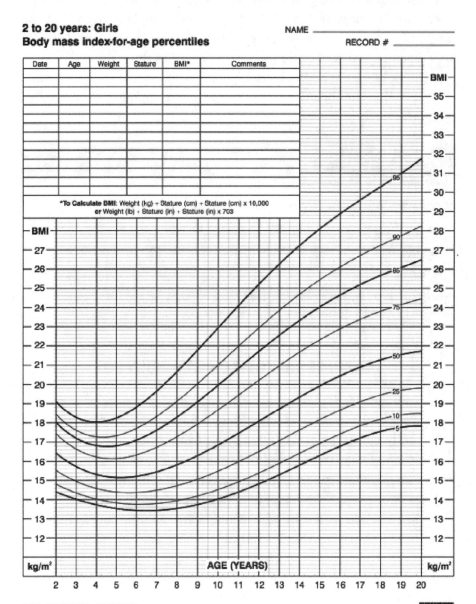

*To Calculate BMI: Weight (kg) ÷ Stature (cm) ÷ Stature (cm) x 10,000
or Weight (lb) ÷ Stature (in) ÷ Stature (in) x 703

Published May 30, 2000 (modified 10/16/00).
SOURCE: Developed by the National Center for Health Statistics in collaboration with
the National Center for Chronic Disease Prevention and Health Promotion (2000).
http://www.cdc.gov/growthcharts

SAFER · HEALTHIER · PEOPLE

To read the stature-for-age and weight-for-age BMI percentile charts for boys (Table 3.4 on page 37) and girls (Table 3.5 on page 38), find your child's height and weight along the left or right side. Follow the straight line to where it intersects with your child's age, listed across the top and bottom. The numbers within the curved lines in the column between ages nineteen and twenty are the BMI percentiles they fall into for their age, based on stature and weight.

See Table 3.6 below for percentile range-defined weight status categories.

TABLE 3.6. WEIGHT CATEGORIES BY PERCENTILE

WEIGHT STATUS CATEGORY*	PERCENTILE RANGE
Underweight	Less than the 5th percentile
Healthy weight	5th percentile to less than the 85th percentile
Overweight	85th to less than the 95th percentile
Obese	Equal to or greater than the 95th percentile

*Standards set by Expert Committee on the Assessment, Prevention, and Treatment of Child and Adolescent Overweight and Obesity: June 6, 2007

DETERMINING YOUR CHILD'S BODY FAT

With an understanding of what BMI is and how it is calculated, parents can have a benchmark by which to determine if their child has a weight problem. But BMI is not the only criteria from which such a determination is made. Other factors need to be taken into account as well, such as waist measurement, fat-to-lean muscle ratio, and other physical characteristics of overweight and obesity in boys and girls.

Waist measurements are easy enough to obtain by simple observations of the numbers on the tape measure, but measuring fat-to-lean muscle ratio is not so visually obvious. It needs to be calculated based on a group of factors that are different in boys and girls. For boys, it encompasses their waist measurement in inches, their weight in pounds, and age in years. For girls, it includes these three factors, plus their wrist, hip, and forearm circumferences in inches.

TABLE 3.4. STATURE-FOR-AGE AND WEIGHT-FOR-AGE BMI PERCENTILES FOR BOYS (AGES 2 TO 20)

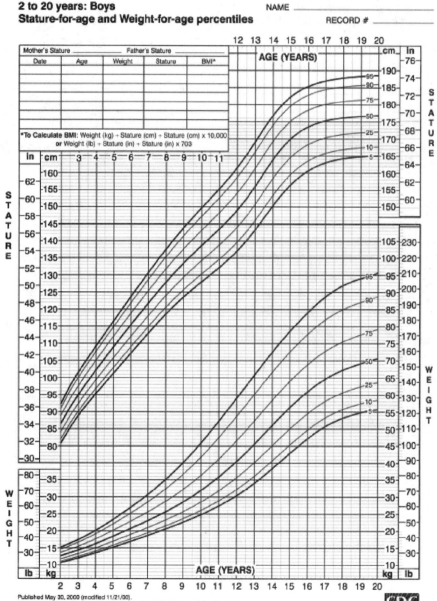

2 to 20 years: Boys
Stature-for-age and Weight-for-age percentiles

NAME _____

RECORD # _____

Published May 30, 2000 (modified 11/21/00).
SOURCE: Developed by the National Center for Health Statistics in collaboration with
the National Center for Chronic Disease Prevention and Health Promotion (2008).
http://www.cdc.gov/growthcharts

SAFER · HEALTHIER · PEOPLE™

TABLE 3.5. STATURE-FOR-AGE AND WEIGHT-FOR-AGE BMI PERCENTILES FOR GIRLS (AGES 2 TO 20)

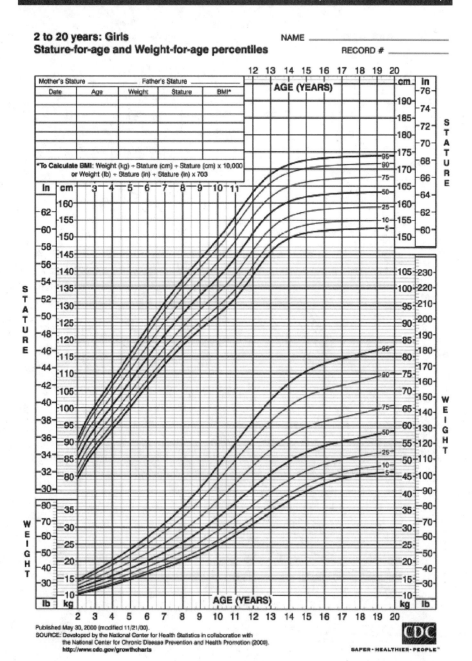

2 to 20 years: Girls
Stature-for-age and Weight-for-age percentiles

NAME

RECORD #

Published May 30, 2000 (modified 11/21/00).
SOURCE: Developed by the National Center for Health Statistics in collaboration with
the National Center for Chronic Disease Prevention and Health Promotion (2000).
http://www.cdc.gov/growthcharts

SAFER·HEALTHIER·PEOPLE™

Keeping track of your child's body fat percentage is a much more useful assessment tool than the scale or the tape measure, especially if they are exercising regularly to lose weight. It is simply the percentage of body weight that consists of fat as opposed to lean muscle. Once you know that, you also know the approximate weight of your child's lean mass (muscle, blood, tissue, etc.) and the approximate weight of their fat.

Again, to make your calculation process easier, here is a link to the Inch-Aweigh.com website (www.inch-aweigh.com/calc_body_fat.htm), where a chart will do the work for you in calculating your child's fat-to-lean muscle ratio. You simply go to the chart, check off whether male or female, enter the numbers requested, then click on "Calculate." The numbers that will appear will show your child's body fat percentage, lean weight (in pounds), and how many pounds of fat they have in their bodies.

See Table 3.7 below for percentile range-defined body fat categories.

TABLE 3.7. BODY FAT PERCENTAGE		
WOMEN	MEN	CATEGORY
10–12%	2–4%	Minimum
14–20%	6–13%	Lean
21–24%	14–17%	Ideal
25–31%	18–25%	Average
> 32%	> 25%	Overweight or Obese

Males with a body fat percentage of 25 percent and above and females with a body fat percentage of 32 percent and above are considered to be "Overweight or Obese." "Average" or "Normal" percentages are between 25 and 31 percent for women, and 18 and 25 percent for men. Between 21 and 24 percent for women and 14 and 17 percent for men is considered "Ideal," and "Lean," the condition generally sought by serious athletes, is between 14 and 20 percent for women, and 6 and 13 percent for men. The "Minimum" amount of body fat to stay alive is between 10 and 12 percent for women, and 2 and 4 percent for men, but this is not considered to be a healthy range for most people.

Other Methods of Measuring Body Fat

There are other, more high-tech methods of measuring body fat, such as hydrostatic weighing and the use of skinfold calipers, but they generally cannot be done at home by the average person. Hydrostatic weighing is a method for determining body composition that involves weighing the body under water. Skinfold calipers are used to measure body fat by pinching the skinfold thickness of many different sites on the body. Your child's pediatrician is the best person to take these kinds of measurements. Please keep in mind that becoming *too* lean is just as unhealthy as becoming overweight, so it's probably wisest to shoot for a number in the "ideal" or "average" category, as described above, depending on your child's current status.

FOR ACCURACY, USE A COMBINATION OF MEASURES

One of the reasons why scale weight alone is no longer used as the measure for overweight or obesity is that the numbers can be misleading. For example, 300 pounds may sound like a lot of weight, and it is; however, if we're talking about a professional football offensive lineman who is also six foot five and in top physical condition, that weight might be standard, when you take into account his fat-to-lean muscle ratio. According to scale weight, your child may seem to be overweight, but because of such factors as their height or fat-to-lean muscle ratio, they may fall within healthy body fat ranges.

All these measurements should be taken into consideration when determining the status of your child's weight. High weight does not always mean high body fat.

With access to the Internet and the links to these websites that calculate BMI and fat-to-lean muscle ratio, parents can chart their kid's progress toward attaining acceptable levels. This should be done as a family so that the child does not feel singled out as an individual. I recommend that this be done on a weekly basis, accompanied by a program of physical activity and healthy eating (detailed in Parts Three and Four) and regular checkups by a doctor. The numbers should be recorded on a journal or diary and compared each week to determine your child's progress or lack of it. (See This Week's Weight in Chapter 10 for tracking your child's progress.) If there has been no progress or a reversal of the numbers from one week to the next, adjustments will likely need to be made to your child's exercise and/or dietary regimen.

A PEDIATRICIAN'S ASSESSMENT

Now, to address the second question posed at the beginning of this chapter: What are some of the danger signs that a child might be overweight or developing a weight problem? For the answer to that question, I turned to the expertise of Dr. Michael Wasserman, my son's pediatrician. Dr. Wasserman, who has been in practice for twenty-seven years and has been featured regularly as an expert on children's health on WWL-TV for the past sixteen years, developed a questionnaire (see page 42) that is designed to alert parents to red flags and symptoms that are causes for concern for their kids.

"Unfortunately, many parents are in denial," Dr. Wasserman asserts. "They tend to ignore what's going on with their kids and choose not to pay attention, but there are some obvious signs they should be alert to." Chief among the signs noted by Dr. Wasserman are clothing sizes worn by their kids. "If they're fitting into larger sizes than would be normal for kids their age that should be a red flag right there."

Dr. Wasserman also cites some other warning signs that a child might be overweight, such as getting fatigued easily, having less stamina, having less ability to engage in even light or moderate exercise, developing low self-esteem, and what he termed the "Pickwickian syndrome," a disorder that was named after Joe, the fat, red-faced boy in Charles Dickens's *The Pickwick Papers*, that involves sleeping problems such as sleep apnea and snoring. "Parents may not see these problems because the child isn't on the football team or the soccer team. They're not seeing these problems because the kids are avoiding that area of their life. They aren't going there," Dr. Wasserman notes.

In some instances in which overweight boys are on the football team precisely because they are overweight, Dr. Wasserman says, "I have a real

QUESTIONNAIRE: PARENTAL RED FLAGS TO CHILDHOOD OBESITY

1. How often does your child eat at restaurants per week?

2. Does your child eat school food for either breakfast or lunch?

3. If your child brings lunch to school, does he/she oftentimes trade foods with others?

4. What do you have to drink in your refrigerator?

    a. Sugared, soft drinks and juices?

    b. Whole (full-fat) milk?

5. What do you have to snack on in your house? How often are snacks eaten?

6. How many portions of fresh fruit and vegetables are consumed daily?

7. Is everyone in the household following the same dietary pattern? Or are there some foods for some adults/children and a different diet for the child with a weight problem?

8. When you eat at home, how many portions does your child eat?

9. Does your child "sneak" food?

10. How often does your child eat at a relative's house (notably grandparents) per week? Do you know the quality of foods, and number and size of portions provided?

11. How many hours daily does your child watch television, play videogames, or spend doing other electronics?

12. How many minutes daily is your child physically active?

13. Is your child relying on a parent's presence to be exercising?

14. Is/are parent(s) good role model(s) by being physically active themselves?

15. Is your child relying on a team sport to be exercising? What does your child do between team seasons?

16. What does your child do during school holidays or summer vacations? Is there daily physical activity involved? Is your child supervised during those times?

17. Is your child more easily fatigued than his/her peers?

18. Has your child's clothes sizes changed?

19. Do you think that your child "has a weight problem"? If so, why? If not, why not?

20. Do you know your child's height, weight, BMI?

Your answers to these questions, if you know what they are, can provide the key to your understanding as to whether or not your child might be overweight and, if so, what issues need to be addressed. Some of these issues you may be able to resolve yourself; others may require professional guidance. Dr. Wasserman suggests that if ten of the questions he poses are answered in "a less than desirable fashion," the child could be at some risk for obesity, and fifteen or more questions, similarly, could put the child at great risk.

problem with that." For many years, high school football coaches have been drafting heavy-set boys onto the team, primarily as offensive linemen where their size is expected to help protect the quarterback and open up holes for running backs. However, many of these overweight boys may not be athletically inclined and, if they're not properly conditioned for the sport, if they're not lean, problems may result.

To determine whether or not a child is overweight or obese, Dr. Wasserman says he starts with the child's BMI—measuring it, charting it, and tracking it regularly. Parents can then do their part by being alert to percentiles, then determining whether or not their child fits into an acceptable range. In some cases, Dr. Wasserman may also request a standard laboratory evaluation that usually includes a lipid profile for measuring cholesterol, a fasting blood sugar (glucose) test, and other tests to measure thyroid levels, insulin levels, and hemoglobin A1c (a protein in red blood cells). These tests, Dr. Wasserman points out, are very effective in determining whether the child has or is at-risk for developing type 2 diabetes and/or cardiovascular disease. If caught soon enough, these conditions may be headed off.

Moderating the child's caloric intake, a regular program of physical exercise, and regular checkups with the child's pediatrician, Dr. Wasserman agrees, are the most effective weapons in the parents' arsenal against their children becoming overweight or obese. He strongly advises parents to cut down on their children's sedentary pursuits ("screen time") and the amount of times they eat out, particularly at fast food outlets. He urges parents to encourage their kids to get out and play more often, and he advocates for healthier meals prepared and consumed at home.

SEE YOUR DOCTOR

OK, so now you've measured and weighed your child and done the assessment. Your verdict is that your child may be overweight. Now what? This next step is critical: *Confirm this with your doctor* or other qualified heathcare professional, so they can recommend a course of action. Before you begin any sort of weight-loss or exercise program, this comes first.

Make an appointment with your family doctor to consult on the proper course of action for your child, yourself, or any other family member contemplating beginning a new fitness or nutrition regimen. Work with your doctor to determine the proper goal weight for your child or yourself. According to Dr. Wasserman, the amount of weight your child should lose depends on how overweight they may be for their particular stage of development. It is generally expected that children will, to use the common expression, "grow into their weight," but this may not always be possible, Dr. Wasserman noted. "For older children who are truly obese—for example, 50 to 100 pounds over ideal weight—it is unlikely that they will grow into their weight, whereas, for toddlers and young children it is more potentially feasible."

This book and others like it can offer only general guidelines and suggestions. But no two people are alike—and no two people can follow exactly the same plan. The safest and best way to achieve your goals is to work with your doctor to determine specific issues and courses of action for you and your child.

WHAT PARENTS CAN DO

With all the great wealth of information out there in cyberspace, it would be impossible for me to list all the useful sources that can help parents educate themselves and their children on issues related to childhood obesity. I list some online sources and websites in the Resources section at the end of this book and you can check them out for yourself. However, one site I find particularly helpful is called Project PACT, (Parents And Children Together), and is sponsored by Revolution Health. As implied by the acronym, it is literally a "pact" between parents and their kids with the common goal of making greater health "a family affair."

On their website, www.revolutionhealth.com/healthy-living/weight-management/special-feature/childhood-obesity, Project PACT offers a four-step guide that will, in their words, "lead your child on a path toward a happier, healthier, thinner, and more fulfilling life." When you visit the site you will see a number of subcategories you can click on for additional, more detailed information. All medical information on this site is peer reviewed.

CHAPTER 3 SUMMARY

- Scale weight can often be misleading due to the fact that it does measure changes in lean muscle, fat and fluid balance.

- By understanding what BMI is and how it is calculated, parents can have a benchmark by which to determine if their child is overweight or obese.

- However, BMI is not the only indicator of the child being over fat, nor should it be used as the determining factor in classifying obesity.

- Scale weight, waist measurements, fat-to-lean muscle ratio, and other physical characteristics should also be used to determine the child's classification of overweight, obesity, or normal weight relative to height, weight, and growth charts.

• Parents should be aware of the potential red flags to childhood obesity and address these issues with the family, child, and doctor, as a team without singling out the overweight child.

CHAPTER 4

Reacting to Insults and Low Self-Esteem

How to Recognize and Manage the Emotional Issues of Your Overweight Child

eing overweight not only has physical ramifications, it carries heavy emotional baggage as well. This can be true for overweight adults, who may be passed over for employment or job promotions, or it may adversely impact them in other types of interactions, even though such discrimination is illegal. It goes on anyway, covertly, and often the person being passed over cannot be certain that their physical size is the reason, even if they strongly suspect it may be so. Intangible factors like these are difficult to prove when no verbal or other physical evidence exists.

If being overweight can pose serious physical and emotional problems for adults, imagine what it must be like for an overweight child. Our Western culture places a premium on physical appearance that goes beyond the health benefits of being slim. Everywhere we look, whether in print, on TV, in the movies, or on the Internet, we see men and women— usually young—who seem to have that "perfect look." The Hollywood or professional model "look." With this "perfect look" being held up as a yardstick, the rest of us are challenged to measure up to it, and often the failure to do so can have serious psychological consequences.

THE SOCIAL AND EMOTIONAL FALLOUT OF BEING OVERWEIGHT

To many people—especially to a child's peers—"looks are everything." As a result, the child who is overweight is often subjected to insults, teasing, ridicule, ostracism, and other offensive remarks. In extreme instances, it can even escalate into physical abuse. Schoolyard bullies sometimes take a perverse delight in beating up on the "fat kids." Kids, as we parents all know from having been there ourselves, can be merciless and unforgiving. They're at an age in which they are becoming increasingly aware of their environment and the world around them, and of other kids their age. If one of their peers deviates from the norm—whether due to a lesser degree of intelligence, physical defects, or other characteristics that single them out—kids will often target those individuals who are "different" from them.

So it is with kids who are overweight. They are particularly susceptible to insults. We all know the broad lexicon of epithets thrown at these overweight boys and girls by others in their age group (and sometimes even by their parents or others who are older), and there is no need to repeat any of them here. New, equally demeaning terms for fatness are entering the kids' vocabulary all the time, all with the same malicious intent and result. And one of those results is potentially serious psychological harm that can become long term. A child can be literally "scarred for life," in other words, well into adulthood, by the emotional abuse heaped upon them because they are fat as youngsters.

In nearly all cases, it is the classic question of "Which came first, the chicken or the egg?" Is the overweight child overeating because he or she is emotionally distressed and has turned to food for comfort and solace, or has he or she developed low self-esteem and/or depression because they don't like their body image?

If an overweight child seems moody or depressed, how serious a problem is it? Is this a short-term condition that will pass, or does the child require counseling, or a psychiatric evaluation? Or, in some instances, prescription medication? For guidance in navigating this sensitive region of a child's growing-up process, I turned to my longtime friend and colleague, Dr. Rob Dahmes, a respected clinical psychiatrist in private practice and clinical assistant professor in the Department of Psychiatry at Louisiana State University, whose expertise comes from many years of counseling kids and their parents.

A CLINICAL PSYCHIATRIST'S OBSERVATIONS

"Obese and overweight children are clearly on the lower end of the social totem pole," according to Dr. Dahmes. He acknowledges that, while obesity may be hereditary in some families, eating practices passed on to children may also be a serious contributing factor. "We know that the laying down of fat cells occurs early on," Dr. Dahmes noted. "Once the fat cell is there, it's there forever. You don't lose fat cells; you lose fat from fat cells. Our society looks at infants as healthy if they have those rosy pink cheeks, and a fat little belly and round bottom." Overfeeding infants, he says, can cause them to be overweight or obese later on, which can lead to psychological as well as physical problems.

Dr. Dahmes spoke of so-called comfort foods, such as cookies, candy, sugary soft drinks, and other sweets that are less than nutritious or high in carbohydrates, that can cause children to become overweight. These comfort foods are often offered by well-intentioned parents or other adults as rewards for good behavior or good grades in school or other similar circumstances in which the child has done well at something. In other instances, especially around holidays, families like to get together and consume large meals. Often families have many pleasant associations with these social gatherings and eating great quantities of rich, starchy, and sweet foods. Many different cultures have a tradition of preparing and enjoying huge meals and encouraging everyone—especially children—to eat. These situations can result in children becoming overweight or obese, and associating these types of foods with comfort and emotional security.

Paraphrasing psychoanalyst Sigmund Freud, Dr. Dahmes noted that the first stage of psychosexual development is oral development. "What he [Freud] was talking about is that there is a great deal of pleasure derived from sensations involving the lips and the mouth, breast-feeding, and so on. If that kind of stimulation gives a great deal of contentment, they (children) continue in that tradition and find a great deal of pleasure in eating.

"When a child turns to food as the primary source of happiness and contentment, it is at the expense of the healthier means of achieving a sense of security," Dr. Dahmes continued. "The child turns away from relationships with significant others, becomes more isolated, and is less focused on school, grades, praise, or accomplishments."

On the subject of depression, Dr. Dahmes says much of it can be attributed to the child's physical appearance, which is often related to their weight and how they are perceived by others, especially their peers. Their feelings of self-worth and self-esteem may suffer and develop into depression.

Dr. Dahmes offers some clues that parents can look for in their kids to help spot depression and gauge its seriousness. Together, the first letters of these clues appropriately spell the phrase "In Sad Cages" as summarized below.

PARENTAL CLUES TO CHILDHOOD DEPRESSION AND DISTRESS

- **IN** = Loss of interest *in* usual activities—A child who, prior to becoming depressed, had lots of interests and enjoyed being active and around other people, might start losing interest in those activities as his or her depression level increases.

- **S** = *Sleep* disturbance—Typically, depressed kids either sleep abnormally long amounts of time, or they may have problems falling asleep. They may also wake up in the middle of the night or earlier than normal in the morning.

- **A** = Changes in *appetite*—With depression you are likely to either see kids with a substantial increase in appetite or a noticeable and possibly unhealthy decrease in their food consumption.

- **D** = *Depressed* mood—When we think of depression most people associate it with being sad and gloomy. With little kids, older kids, and teenagers they can be sad and gloomy, but they can also be irritable, easily frustrated, or ill tempered.

- **C** = Poor *concentration* and memory—Grades start to fall in school because the kids aren't paying as much attention as they once did.

- **A** = Change in level of physical *activity*—Depressed kids typically begin to slow down, become less active than they were. They become "couch potatoes," planting themselves in front of the TV or computer, or pursuing other solitary, sedentary activities.

- **G** = *Guilt* and low self-esteem—Kids and adolescents who are depressed often feel guilty about minor things, and this can result in low self-esteem. They may feel they're too fat, too skinny, too small, too stupid, or too smart. Whatever the case may be, they are not happy with who they are.

- **E** = *Energy* levels—Kids and adolescents who are depressed may be experiencing excessive levels of fatigue.

- **S** = Thoughts of *suicide*. Though this is largely applicable to older children and teenagers, it can be a serious problem among eight to twelve-year-olds as well. In fact, suicide is the third leading cause of death in children and adolescents. When a depressed child says something like, "I wish I was dead" or "I think I'll kill myself," they should be taken seriously. Many youngsters have, unfortunately, made good on those words. Regarding the last category, Dr. Dahmes noted that, to protect families in cases of kids taking too many antidepressants, coroners will sometimes list cause of death as being "accidental overdoses" when, in fact, they may have actually been suicides.

"The most effective means of determining the seriousness of depression is rating the degree of impairment in the day-to-day functioning of the child or adolescent. This includes social, behavioral, physical, and cognitive functioning," Dr. Dahmes added. As a means of grading degrees of depression, using the In Sad Cages model, he suggests assigning a zero to a behavior if it is absent or a numeral 1 if the behavior is present. If the total score is 0 to 3, depression would be considered mild or minimal. A score of 4 to 7 would be considered moderate, and an 8 or above would be severe, necessitating immediate professional attention.

As a clinical psychiatrist, Dr. Dahmes noted that "You can't just treat a child who's depressed with medication alone. It is only one component of an arsenal of interventions that may be called upon to treat the depressed child or adolescent. Other effective methods of treatment include behavioral counseling, individual psychotherapy, group psychotherapy, and family therapy.

"You have to make lifestyle changes, as well," Dr. Dahmes continued. "Parental dynamics have to be addressed. A multi-modal, multi-faceted approach has to be taken. Even though parents may have busy, active careers and lifestyles, they can't just take the easy way out and pick up fast food on the way home to feed their kids."

Dr. Dahmes noted the role parents may inadvertently play in whether or not their kids are overweight. For example, if the parents are frequently fighting and arguing, this can traumatize a child and cause them to seek comfort and relief in something that is pleasurable to them, such as eating. And what they're eating may not be the healthiest things for them, and this can contribute to their weight problem. "So, in addition to modeling appropriate eating patterns, parents also have to model appropriate anger management, conflict resolution, and discussion. If the parents exercise, that too, can be an appropriate model for the kids to emulate," Dr. Dahmes said.

OTHER PSYCHOLOGICAL REPERCUSSIONS OF BEING OVERWEIGHT

Other findings also appear to pinpoint some of the psychological problems overweight and obese children may endure.

IQ and Learning

According to a study published in the *Journal of Pediatrics* (August 2006), children who are very obese by the age of four may be more likely to have lower IQ scores. The team conducting the study of eighteen people who had been morbidly obese by age four and a comparable number of their siblings who weren't, showed an average gap of 25 to 30 points on the IQ scale. Those who had Prader-Willi syndrome (a rare but commonly rec-ognized genetic cause of childhood obesity that is also linked to mental retardation), and others who had early morbid obesity, scored much lower than those who were not morbidly obese in early childhood.

Doctors involved in conducting the study were not certain what the connection might be between early childhood obesity and intelligence, but they concluded that "the first few years of life are a critical time for brain development." During the study, those who were eleven years of age and older were given brain scans using magnetic resonance imaging (MRI). Children who had been morbidly obese by age four were observed as having white spots on different regions of their brains. These white spots were not understood by those conducting the study, and further research is needed to interpret them. However, as one of the doctors conducting the study observed, "They are not a good thing." These white spots could very well be linked to gaps in these children's range of intelligence.

Another study made public about a month later showed that girls who became overweight between the time they started kindergarten and fin-ished the third grade suffered a decline in test scores and social skills, and scored lower than girls who were not overweight. But boys who gained weight in their early school years suffered far fewer negative conse-quences than girls in the same age group. The study measured test results in math and reading skills, as well as teacher-reported externalized behav-ior problems, and teacher ratings of interpersonal skills and approaches to learning.

Some of the factors regarding intelligence that need to be taken into account, Dr. Dahmes noted, may be the child's family's socioeconomic background. Many of these families might not be able to afford the con-tinuously rising prices on some of the healthier types of foods—primari-ly fruits and vegetables. Also, if the child is coming from a home in which learning and studying are not strongly encouraged, this may very well be reflected in that child's level of intelligence or their ability or willingness to learn.

The bottom line is this: if a child's intelligence level is significantly lower than that of his or her peers, not only might it affect their personalities by making them feel inferior, but it could also subject them to psychologically damaging insults from their peers. These findings, like those from other similar studies, appear to point to serious psychological problems experienced by kids at an early age. These problems often spill over into adulthood.

Eating Disorders

Although eating disorders such as anorexia nervosa, bulimia nervosa, and binge eating disorders are more of a problem for older kids and adolescents, they may be rooted in problems that began in early childhood. Even though kids with these conditions are generally not overweight or obese, they may *think* they are. In trying to live up to unrealistic standards of body weight expectation, many of them run the risk of developing one of these eating disorders—especially teenage girls who are competing for boys with other girls their age. Recent studies show that 90 percent of those diagnosed with anorexia nervosa are female.

Kids with anorexia nervosa are possessed by an overriding and often unrealistic fear of gaining weight: they think they are fat but they're not. Self-starvation is the primary cause. The youngster not only fears they are gaining weight, but they also may have an unrealistic image of themselves and how they think they should look. This can cause serious psychological harm, in that the youngster may feel like a failure if he or she doesn't measure up to a physical appearance standard that may be unattainable.

Bulimia nervosa is an eating disorder that involves binge eating and then attempting to purge all or most of what was consumed. The person experiencing it may try to force themselves to vomit, or they may use laxatives, or they may indulge in excessive exercising in order to disgorge what they've eaten. Binge eating disorder is largely the same as bulimia, with the difference being that the child doesn't attempt to purge what they ate.

Anorexia, especially, has received a great deal of publicity in recent years because a number of young, high-profile film and music stars have been diagnosed with it. A few have even died from it. The most high-profile case was that of singer Karen Carpenter whose death at a young age in 1983 brought anorexia nervosa to the attention of the world. Children and teens diagnosed with anorexia have a 5 to 7 percent chance of dying within ten years, and those with bulimia may die within five years from their disease or suicide related to it.

Anorexia, bulimia, and binge eating disorders are serious concerns and they must be dealt with realistically once they are diagnosed. Dr. Dahmes notes, "They are very difficult conditions to deal with, but they can be effectively treated with early and consistent interventions. Although they share strong psychological components, there does appear to be some genetic influences in these disorders as well." However, he is quick to note that the genetic component—which can't be altered—does not appear to be as strong as the psychological components, which can be altered.

Studies appear to be showing that, if treated properly, a person with an eating disorder has a 70 percent chance of recovery. A proper diet and regular exercise regimen can accomplish the same results—or better—than starving or gorging then purging oneself. However, before such conditions can develop in a child's adolescent years, the potential for such conditions should be caught in their earlier years, and professionals who work with these types of problems strongly believe it can be done.

Parents who are concerned about whether or not their kids either have or may be prone to having eating disorders can obtain more information by going to the appropriate websites listed in the Resources section of this book.

WHAT PARENTS CAN DO

Many books and journal articles have been devoted to the subject of helping kids cope with such diverse stressors as bullying, peer pressure, violence, drugs, and other negative factors. However, for "concrete steps" for parents to remember in helping their children and adolescents to cope, Dr. Dahmes offers the following advice:

- Be available to openly discuss and communicate.

- Practice consistency and predictability in dealing with problems and crises.

- Be absolutely honest and practice what you preach.

- Always encourage personal responsibility and self-confidence.

- Always be a parent, not a friend, big brother, or big sister.

In addition, it's important for parents to remember to reward and reinforce positive eating and lifestyle behaviors in children. They need to model the behaviors they wish their kids to adopt. Parents will get better results with using positive language—encouraging kids to adopt a healthier lifestyle rather than criticizing, blaming, or using pejorative expressions that may further exacerbate the problem. Parents need to build and enforce emotional strength and self-esteem in kids so that they are motivated to make better choices.

CHAPTER 4 SUMMARY

- Being overweight not only has physical ramifications, it carries heavy emotional baggage as well, especially for children.

- Parents should be aware of early signs of depression and early distress in their child by using the phrase "In Sad Cages" and respond to these cues immediately.

- Parents should also learn to recognize the early signs of eating disorders.

- Parent should strive to create a healthy, stable, and low-stress home environment and help the child learn to cope with emotional issues in a healthy manner, as a part of an overall family positive lifestyle plan.

PART THREE

The Nutritional
Body Plan

CHAPTER 5

Beyond Dieting

Building a Healthier Relationship with Food

Good nutrition starts at home and lasts a lifetime. The benefits of eating right as a family include not only developing good nutritional habits in kids, but also laying down the foundations for a strong and healthy body they will hopefully carry for the rest of their lives. If a child does not get proper nutrition and stay physically active during the crucial years of childhood (especially between the ages of eight and twelve when the body is maturing), then their organ systems, immune system, and metabolism may not develop properly.

As you've learned, when a child becomes overweight or obese, there is the added threat of developing serious illnesses at a young age. Even if these illnesses are not contracted in the child's early years, the groundwork may be laid for their development later on. However, it is difficult to motivate kids to eat right by warning them about long-term health problems such as heart disease, kidney disease, elevated levels of bad cholesterol, hypertension (high blood pressure), and type 2 diabetes. Adult health issues are difficult concepts for youngsters to grasp. At their young ages, kids tend to think they will always be youthful and energetic, and will never be susceptible to the disorders their parents and other older adults may suffer from.

For these reasons, parents need a practical plan for countering their child's resistance to eating correctly. Parents must empower and strongly encourage their child to begin making healthier choices. In so doing, parents who are in denial about their child's weight have to overcome that denial and face the problem realistically.

As touched upon earlier, a *Consumer Reports* survey of more than 3,000 parents taken in 2007 showed that roughly 50 percent of those surveyed felt that their child was not overweight even when their kid's BMI indicated otherwise. A large part of the problem, the study noted, had to do with food issues; that is, the types of foods that parents are feeding their children. If the parents are not aware of the carbohydrate and fat content of the foods they're putting on their child's plate, the child isn't going to know either. Kids will eat what's in front of them without realizing that it might be contributing to their weight problem.

A HEALTHY APPROACH TO WEIGHT LOSS

Many parents hope that their overweight child will simply "grow out of their baby fat" as they get older. Unfortunately, if a child continues to have poor eating habits and low activity levels, it is highly likely that the problem will only get worse. Yet, putting kids on a calorie-restrictive diet is not the answer. It can actually be *un*healthy. Since children are growing, they *need* a certain amount of calories and a variety of healthy foods on a daily basis to keep their bodies growing properly and to prevent deficiencies. Also, imposing food restrictions on children and making them "go hungry" can sometimes lead to eating disorders later in life. The best approach to helping an overweight or obese child reach a normal weight is to create balanced nutritional patterns that will teach them to *manage* their weight so that they can literally become leaner as they grow.

According to a 1990 report by the Education Resources Information Center (ERIC, formerly the Office of Educational Research and Improvement Clearinghouse) on Teaching and Teacher Education, "Obesity treatment programs for children and adolescents rarely have weight loss as a goal. Rather, the aim is to slow or halt weight gain so the child will grow into his or her body weight over a period of months to years." Quoting from a 1983 article by pediatrician W. H. Dietz in the *Journal of Pediatrics,* the ERIC report goes on to estimate that for every 20 percent excess of ideal body weight, the child will need one and a half years of weight maintenance to attain ideal body weight." When a child's metabolism is fueled correctly through healthier nutritional habits—and stimulated properly through higher levels of activity—children naturally begin to lose weight as they grow.

It is a challenge getting kids to stop eating junk food when many of them are addicted to the sugary and salty flavors and the good feelings they get from comfort foods. For some guidance to these issues I consulted registered dietitian Julie Fortenberry, my nutritionist at The Fitness Principle with Mackie Shilstone. As Julie explains, it is certainly possible, with patience and perseverance and by offering equally enjoyable alternatives, to offer a new paradigm for family nutrition and effective strategies for helping kids develop better eating habits. Here is what she had to say on adding some variety and basic nutrition to children's diets.

A NUTRITIONIST'S PERSPECTIVE

"One of the biggest problems I see with kids is getting them to try new things. They're picky eaters," Julie notes. "They've gotten into a routine of convenient foods from childhood, and these convenient foods are usually high-calorie, intensely sweet or salty, products. Getting them to try a new fruit, a new vegetable, or a new meat is a big challenge. Many parents just give up and let them eat the same things they've always been eating." And much of what they've always eaten may not be the healthiest things for them. Julie suggests some alternatives.

"Parents need to work with their kids and stay patient with them, encouraging them to try new things but not forcing them," Julie says. She suggests putting spinach on their plate with one of their favorite foods like macaroni and cheese, or something else they really enjoy. "If they don't eat everything, just take the plate away and do not make it a big deal. Eventually, the kids may come to like something they were initially averse to. Maybe after fifteen or twenty times they'll decide they like it," she says. "It takes patience, encouragement, and understanding to develop new habits."

Julie also noted that kids have a natural ability to know when they've eaten enough. Babies will turn their heads away when they're full, but often the parent doing the feeding will force them to eat more. This, she says, teaches them as children to always eat what is on their plate, whether they are full or not. This can develop into a habit that can result in a child becoming overweight or obese later on. She calls this the "Clean Your Plate Club," and discourages parents from following that line of thinking. She also discourages parents from using analogies with other cultures when trying to get them to eat everything on their plate. "They may say that people are starving in other countries, but we have a problem with obesity in our country which is just as dangerous. We've got to encourage kids to finish eating when they feel pleasant."

The problem, Julie cites, isn't always the quantity or portion sizes of what kids have been eating, it's what they're actually eating in general which, she says, may lack variety or be high-calorie itself. "They're eating foods that are high in calories all or most of the time, as opposed to just every now and then." For example, some children may eat five slices of pizza daily instead of a more moderate and practical two slices a month. Portion sizes are important in relation to what type of food the kids are eating. She recommends smaller portions of the foods highest in fat and sugar content (fried foods, pizza, sodas, etc.) and larger portions of healthy foods like fruit and vegetables. Kids may also have larger portions of meat dishes, as long as the meat is lean or extra lean.

Although parents' main objectives should be to partially wean their kids off foods that are high in fat and sugar content, Julie acknowledges that it is a delicate balance. "They're kids and they often need as many or sometimes even more calories than adults, because they're still growing and developing. The focus should be on good-quality calories, not frequent junk. You don't want to deprive them of anything, because as soon as they leave your sight they're going to eat it, whether it's trading food at school or eating at a friend's house. You don't want to deny them an occasional treat, but you do want to inform them on why you're choosing the healthier choices."

Kids appear to be more receptive to incentives that appeal to their vanity, and physical appearance (for example, clear skin, healthy hair and nails, good vision, etc.), more so than to references to physical conditions that may or may not occur later in life. Explain to them that food is your body's gasoline. If you are putting bad "fuel" into your "car" then it is not going to run properly. Talk to them about "good fuel" (whole grains, fruits, vegetables, etc.) and "bad fuel" (sodas, cookies, chips, etc.). The bad fuel should be limited for the best performance today and long term.

With music lessons, ball practice, play rehearsal, and work schedules, it can be tough to get the family all together at the dinner table. Rounding up the troops for an evening meal can be almost impossible! However, research is beginning to show that eating as a family has great benefits for your children and teenagers. According to a survey conducted by the University of Minnesota that appears in the August 2004 issue of *The Archives of Pediatrics & Adolescent Medicine*, frequent family meals are related to better nutritional intake, and a decreased risk for unhealthy weight control practices and substance abuse. Another University of Minnesota study published in the *Journal of the American Dietetic Association* found that children who ate family meals consumed more fruits and vegetables and fewer snack foods than children who ate separately from their families. It may take some finagling, some rearranging of schedules, and some tenacity on everyone's part, but those who have made the effort and succeeded have found that the rewards made it well worth their while.

A large part of correcting the problem, in many cases, lies with the schools, where kids typically spend up to six or seven hours a day, nine to ten months of the year. If the schools aren't offering healthy food choices for the kids, the kids aren't normally going to go outside the box and demand better quality. This is where parental involvement comes in. Concerned parents in various parts of the country have banded together and put pressure on school boards and individual schools themselves, demanding and receiving healthier food choices from the cafeterias of their kids' schools. In some instances, parental pressure has resulted in the removal of carbonated soft drink machines and candy dispensing machines and replaced them with vending machines that sell only healthy drinks and healthy snacks.

However, the schools themselves need to take some initiatives and not wait for pressure to be put on them by parents. In a statement released by the American Heart Association (AHA) in October 2004, the AHA recommended that schools serve "heart healthy" meals and engage in some type of nutrition education. They also recommended mandatory physical education from kindergarten to grade twelve.

Julie recommends that parents get a copy of their kids' school menus in advance so they can plan lunches together. If the school is offering something that is not so healthy on a particular day and the kids are in agreement with it, parents and kids can then pack along a more nutritious meal for the kids to bring in.

"The reality is, as an eight-year-old, you're going to have unhealthy options for the rest of your life. You're going to have to learn to pick, on those days, healthier choices," Julie says. "Temptations and unhealthy habits are everywhere. You have to encourage your child to make healthy choices."

Parents and children can be misled from making wise food choices by their own lack of product knowledge and common misconceptions. For example, for parents who don't know how to measure portion size, Julie recommends that they use familiar objects to make those types of associations. For example, a serving of fruit might be the size of a baseball, a serving of rice the size of a golf ball (one-third cup), a serving of pasta the size of a tennis ball (one-half cup), a serving of cheese equivalent to a few dice, and a serving of meat the size of a pack of cards. There is a common misconception, she notes, for people to think that what is on a plate or in a package or a can is a serving size. Packages and cans often contain more than one serving, and most restaurant servings should be cut into fourths, Julie says. Also, recommended serving sizes will vary according to each child's needs as determined by such factors as their age, height, weight, and level of activity. (To learn more about apportioning the correct serving sizes for your child, see Table 5.1 on page 69; see also the resources listed at the end of the chapter.)

Julie notes that whether rice, bread, or pasta is white or the healthier whole-grain, high-fiber type, they carry the same amount of calories. She strongly suggests that parents and older kids learn how to read and interpret the Nutrition Facts panel listed on most packaged products. Observe how many "Total Calories" and "Calories from Fat" are in each serving, then note how many grams of fats, carbohydrates, proteins, and other components—including vitamins—are in each serving. (For more on how to read and interpret the Nutrition Facts on food labels, see the resources listed at the end of the chapter.)

In regard to sugar, Julie agrees that natural sugar contained in fresh fruits and honey is healthier for us; however, it is not calorie free. There is another misconception that eating unlimited fruit and drinking more 100 percent fruit juice will help with weight loss. Not so, Julie emphasizes. "They can still contribute to weight gain if you're not careful," she says. Whole fruits and 100 percent juice are full of great nutrients that our bodies need, but we still need to be aware of portions when consuming them. Keep in mind when choosing a product, that ingredients are listed on the product label in descending order by weight. The main ingredient is listed first, followed by other ingredients used in lesser amounts. "So, if the first few items you see on an ingredient list are sugar, high-fructose corn syrup, sucrose, glucose, or even honey, these products are full of sugar. These foods should be limited. You need to limit those types of things. Foods with high-sugar content," she adds, "can lead to cavities in the teeth as well as to obesity."

A general rule to follow when trying to tell if the food you're about to buy is truly healthy or not is to look at the number of ingredients listed on the product label. A product with a lengthy ingredients list is usually a sign that the product has unnecessary extras such as additives, preservatives, and other ingredients with chemical-sounding names, and is the least healthy for you. It is also a good idea to look for food items that contain a lot of vitamins, minerals, and other healthy nutrients like folic acid or calcium. Food supplements, Julie says, can help make up for the nutrients the kids may not be getting from the foods they eat. If the child is not eating a variety of nutritious foods, has food allergies, or is a picky eater, a good multivitamin would be encouraged as a backup source. However, she strongly emphasizes that supplements should not take the place of healthy eating. They don't replace proper nutrition. Parents must continue to offer their children healthy meals and snacks. She also suggests that parents consult with their doctors on which vitamins might be best for their child's individual needs.

For beverage choices, "I usually push water and milk," Julie says, adding that sodas or juices should be limited to no more than two times a week. In addressing these issues, Julie says, "Don't take away all of your kid's favorite foods. Instead, create more nutritional versions of the things they love to eat." She suggests healthy pizza with less cheese and more vegetables and lean meat, or sweet potato french fries that are baked instead of fried in oil. Serve them turkey burgers on whole-wheat or multi-grain buns instead of fatty beef burgers on a white bun, and baked and breaded white-meat chicken strips instead of deep-fried chicken nuggets. These are just a few examples of alternatives parents might want to consider feeding their kids. (For more ideas, see the recipes in Chapter 6.)

However, the development of healthy eating habits also needs to extend beyond the home. Many parents these days may be too busy or too tired to cook every night of the week, so they take their kids out to eat. Once they are in a restaurant, especially a fast food restaurant, measuring portion sizes and regulating nutrition content is largely out of their hands. But it is still possible to eat healthy and the right amount in these environments. Here are some tips suggested by Julie for your family to eat healthier when you're out:

- **Mind the beverages.** Kids' menus often offer a free soda with every entrée. This can add hundreds of calories without adding any nutrition to the meal. Ask for a substitution like water or low-fat milk for the soda.

- **Ask for a different side dish.** While many restaurants do not list any side dish other than french fries, most will allow you to substitute something healthier, like cooked vegetables, sliced tomatoes, or a side salad if you ask.

- **Think outside the kids' section.** Adult menus almost universally offer healthy options. Consider sharing an entrée like grilled chicken or fish with your child, or ask about ordering a half portion or lunch portion. Give your children a few choices and have them pick one. This gives them independence while teaching them examples of healthy foods.

- **Avoid high-fat condiments** such as sour cream, mayonnaise, sauces, and butter. Ask for these items on the side so that you can control your portions.

Overall, though, you should try to limit eating out to no more than twice a week, and when you do eat out, choose restaurants that you know have healthy choices. If your children see that eating out three or more times a week is a family routine, it may be hard for them to change that trend when they are older and making their own choices. An occasional outing to the fast food restaurant may be difficult to avoid, but try not to make it a way of life.

MORE TOOLS FOR DEVELOPING BETTER EATING HABITS

The Weight-control Information Network (WIN), a program sponsored by the National Institute of Diabetes and Digestive and Kidney Diseases, also cites some important guidelines parents should encourage their children to follow. In addition to teaching them healthy eating practices and offering them foods that are higher in nutritional value and lower in fat/sugar content, WIN encourages parents to seek professional advice from doctors and nutritionists. They say that children should never be put on a restrictive weight-loss diet unless supervised for medical reasons by a doctor. They also stress that parents follow the nutrition and serving size guidelines established by the United States Department of Agriculture (USDA) in the Food Pyramid (see Figure 5.1 on page 68).

Using the Food Pyramid

Parents can use the Food Pyramid to help them cultivate a daily pattern of wise food choices—ranging from liberal consumption of grain products, as represented in the first band of the pyramid, to sparing use of meat and beans, as represented in the last band—as well as how many daily servings to eat from each major food group.

The serving sizes listed beneath each food group of the Food Pyramid are for children and adults, two years or older. The smaller number in the serving range is for children who consume about 1,300 calories a day, such as kids two to four years of age. The larger number in the serving range is for those who consume about 3,000 calories a day, such as boys fifteen to eighteen years of age.

FIGURE 5.1. USDA FOOD PYRAMID

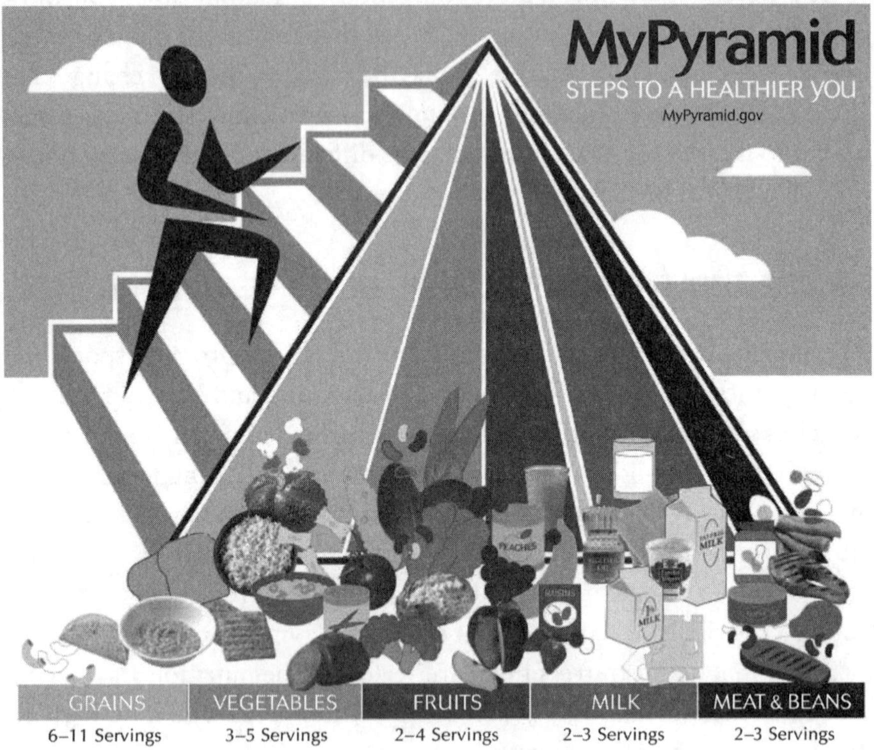

MyPyramid
STEPS TO A HEALTHIER YOU
MyPyramid.gov

GRAINS	VEGETABLES	FRUITS	MILK	MEAT & BEANS
6–11 Servings	3–5 Servings	2–4 Servings	2–3 Servings	2–3 Servings

SOURCE: U.S. Department of Agriculture.

On the opposite page, Table 5.1 provides several examples of what a serving size equals in each food group. Here are some visual ways to picture a serving size using everyday objects.

- A serving of fruit should be about the size of a baseball.

- A serving of rice should be about the size of a golf ball ($1/3$ cup).

- A serving of pasta should be about the size of a tennis ball ($1/2$ cup).

- A baked potato should be about the size of a computer mouse.

- A serving of cheese should be about the size of a few dice.

- A serving of meat should be about the size of a deck of cards.

TABLE 5.1. WHAT DOES A SERVING SIZE EQUAL?

MILK, YOGURT, AND CHEESE (2–3 SERVINGS)

- 1 cup of milk or yogurt
- 1.5 ounces of natural cheese
- 2 ounces of processed cheese

MEAT, POULTRY, FISH, DRY BEANS, EGGS, AND NUTS (2–3 SERVINGS)

- 2–3 ounces of cooked lean meat, poultry, or fish
- $\frac{1}{2}$ cup of cooked dry beans, 1 egg, or 2 tablespoons of peanut butter count as 1 ounce of lean meat

VEGETABLES (3–5 SERVINGS)

- 1 cup of raw leafy vegetables
- $\frac{1}{2}$ cup of other vegetables, cooked or chopped raw
- $\frac{3}{4}$ cup of vegetable juice

FRUITS (2–4 SERVINGS)

- 1 medium apple, banana, orange
- $\frac{1}{2}$ cup of chopped, cooked, or canned fruit
- $\frac{3}{4}$ cup of fruit juice

BREAD, CEREAL, RICE, AND PASTA (6–11 SERVINGS)

- 1 slice of bread
- 1 ounce of ready-to-eat cereal
- $\frac{1}{2}$ cup of cooked cereal, rice, or pasta

Teaching Smart Food Choices

Kids between the ages of eight and twelve still listen to their parents, but during this developmental period they are also actively learning how to make their own choices in life. Many of these choices are the result of pressures put on them by their peers, as well as attitudes they pick up from the media. Advertising is a very powerful medium for getting kids (and adults, also) to consume products that might not be the best for them nutritionally. The more hours they spend in front of a TV set, the more they are bombarded with these types of ads. The American Academy of Pediatrics, in December 2006, approximated that the average American child watches about 40,000 ads a year on TV alone—not counting other media such as magazines they frequently read or websites popular with kids of varying age groups.

To counter this, experts are recommending that kids become much more consumer savvy at younger ages. Children need to analyze food advertisements on their favorite programs more carefully now because of recent increases in additives and preservatives to foods that make them less healthy. It isn't an easy task to accomplish. From the early days of television to the present, many kids' shows have been sponsored by major food companies that offer products that are high in sugar and unhealthy fats. Some groups, such as the American Academy of Pediatrics, have advocated banning junk food ads from children's programming but such bans might not hold up to legal challenges. The Children's Advertising Review Unit of the Council of Better Business Bureaus strongly recommends educating children on consumer issues as they relate to product information.

"Children will be faced with choices in the marketplace their entire lives," notes Arthur Pober, EdD, vice president of the Children's Advertising Review Unit and a specialist in early childhood education. "In order to empower them to become judicious consumers, we must give them the tools to make choices regarding the advertising message and the product." Parents need to be very much a part of this process, Dr. Pober adds, "involving children as young as four years old in decisions about family purchases."

Children can also be misled by their own lack of product knowledge. As Julie pointed out earlier in the chapter, children may think they're drinking something healthy because it's called "fruit drink" but, without checking the ingredient list carefully they may be getting little or no actual fruit content. Many drinks are "fruit flavored" and artificially colored to look like the particular fruit, but they are also high in sugar content and calories and low in nutritional content. And, as is very often the case, parents themselves may be confused by the terms on juice labels and are unaware that they're not buying the healthiest products for their kids. A 1998 survey of pediatricians by the Gallup Organization appeared to confirm this.

Another study, this one announced by the American Psychiatric Association at their annual meeting in May 2005, linked caffeine in carbonated soft drinks—mostly colas—to behavioral problems in kids, in addition to increases in obesity and other health concerns.

Because kids are at or getting to an age where they begin asserting their independence, they are likely to balk at being nagged or *told* what to eat. It is a much more effective strategy to include kids in the process of developing better eating habits by making it a family project. Parents can actively involve kids in making family food choices by giving them a chance to select new recipes, make out a grocery list, and participate in food shopping. They can even help with the preparation of food, which teaches them not only what types of food are good for them, but also how to cook it.

Julie feels it is a good idea to give kids two healthy food choices and let them decide between the two. Ask them if they want a turkey sandwich or a lean ham sandwich, or if they want spinach or eggplant. Don't make it a *multiple* choice or they're liable to make a bad selection. On the other hand, if parents are trying to wean kids off sugary desserts and onto fresh fruits, then it is best to give them several choices of fruits, not just an apple. These fruits should be washed and clearly visible in a basket in the kitchen or family room. If they're in plain sight the kids are more likely to take them than if they're hidden away in the crisper drawers of the refrigerator.

WHAT PARENTS CAN DO

For many parents on the lower end of the economic scale, eating healthy can be expensive. It is a well-known fact that health food stores charge more for their products than conventional supermarkets. However, there are still many products within the price range of most working parents that are healthy, not just for their kids but for them as well. There are a number of reputable, peer-reviewed websites that contain important, easy-to-understand information about how to read product labels, how to determine healthy portion sizes, how to shop for the healthiest products. Listed below are just a few of these sites:

- www.kidshealth.org/parent/nutrition_fit/nutrition/food_labels.html contains information on how to read and interpret Nutrition Facts on food labels;

- www.kidshealth.org/parent/nutrition_fit/nutrition/pyramid.html discusses the Food Guide Pyramid and how to approximate correct portion sizes for your child;

- www.kidshealth.org/parent/food/general/food_shopping.html and www.diabetes.org/for-parents-and-kids/diabetes-care/healthy-eating.jsp offer helpful advice on food shopping with your kids, meal and snack planning, an eating out guide and other helpful tips to get your kids (and you) eating right.

There is even a website that rates the nutritional value of snacks kids commonly eat. It's called the Snackwise Nutrition Rating System. Go to www.nationwidechildrens.org/gd/applications/snackwise/home.cfm.

All you have to do, after you pull up the site, is take a look at any snack product and type in the package information requested in a questionnaire, click on the "Submit" button, and it automatically calculates a rating for you. The ratings are color-coded in green (best choice), yellow (choose occasionally), and red (choose rarely). Try it. I did and it really works!

Remember, nutritional changes can't just involve children but must include the whole family. Since parents are role models for their kids, they must actively make a commitment to eating more nutritionally themselves. In the next chapter, Julie Fortenberry and I share some healthy recipes and food choice recommendations that can lead to healthier meals and healthier eating habits for the entire family.

CHAPTER 5 SUMMARY

- Proper nutrition is essential in maintaining a healthy weight.

- Appropriate nutrition guidelines should be recognized early in the child's life so that good habits can be established long term.

- Parents must strongly encourage and empower their children to make healthy food choices to prevent future health or weight issues.

- Portion sizes are just as important as the food choices they are making.

- Sugar intake from candy, sodas, cookies, cakes, etc., should be limited.

- Learning to read nutrition labels and the product's ingredient list can aid in making a healthy food selection.

CHAPTER 6

Recipes Kids Love

Healthy and Fun Foods to Boost Your Child's Metabolism

E ating right is one of the keys to an effective weight loss plan. There are many types of foods and meal plans that can help accomplish this goal, and in this chapter you will find a few suggestions among the many options that are available. The recipes in this chapter come from my nutritionist at The Fitness Principle with Mackie Shilstone, Julie Fortenberry, plus a few from one of my previous books, *The Fat-Burning Bible* (John Wiley & Sons, 2005).

We have included a few sample selections of healthy foods you can prepare for your child for breakfast, lunch, supper, and snacks in-between meals. While we don't specifically advocate taking away your child's favorite foods, we strongly urge parents to gently guide their kids toward foods that are both healthy for them and as pleasant tasting as those foods they may be giving up. For example, baking potatoes or chicken is healthier for them (and you) than deep-frying them. Substituting whole-wheat bread or pasta for white bread or pasta is also healthier. Once kids get used to alternatives like these, they may find that they actually taste better. There are many things you can do to make their meals healthier without sacrificing taste.

All the dishes presented in this chapter consist of healthy carbohydrates, lean protein, and unsaturated fats. Healthy carbohydrates provide a good source of energy for long days; protein stabilizes blood sugar while making the body feel satiated after a meal; and unsaturated fats improve heart function and help prevent heart disease.

Parents are also encouraged to steer their child toward beverages like water and low-fat milk that are healthier for them than soft drinks and artificially sweetened beverages. Overall, they contain the fewest calories and are the healthiest among the many drink choices kids have.

Note: the recipes in this chapter are not calorie specific. Portion sizes will vary according to the child. Parents of overweight or obese children should always consult with their child's physician and, whenever possible, with a licensed nutritionist for advice on the best foods, meal plans, and portion sizes for their children.

BREAKFAST

Start the day with a good breakfast. It really is the most important meal of the day. It wakes up your brain and body! Don't have time? Try these quick breakfast ideas.

- Whole-wheat bread and peanut butter

- Whole-wheat bread and a boiled egg (boil the night before)

- Whole-wheat bread and lean deli meat

- Pack of plain oatmeal with a scoop of peanut butter

- Pack of grits made with 2 percent cheese (any kind)

- Whole-wheat English muffin with 2 percent cheese and turkey or Canadian bacon

Here are some more healthy breakfast recipes for you and your kids.

BERRY GOOD MUFFINS

YIELD: 12 MUFFINS

1 cup whole-grain flour

1 cup quick-cooking oatmeal

1 teaspoon salt

4 teaspoons baking powder

1 cup blueberries, washed

1 egg

1 cup skim or 1 percent milk

¼ cup canola oil

Nonstick spray or paper liners

Preheat the oven to 400°F. In a large bowl, mix together the flour, oatmeal, salt, and baking powder. Gently fold in the blueberries. In another bowl, break the egg and use a fork to beat it just a little bit. Then add the milk and vegetable oil, and mix. When well combined, add this mixture to the dry ingredients in the large bowl. Using a mixing spoon, mix about 25 or 30 times. Don't mix too much! Your muffin mixture should be lumpy, not smooth.

Next line a twelve-cup muffin tin with paper liners or lightly spray with nonstick spray. Spoon in the muffin mix. Fill each muffin cup about two-thirds of the way up. Bake for about 20 minutes. When the muffins are finished baking, remove them from the muffin tin and cool them on a wire rack. Enjoy!

ZUCCHINI MUFFINS

YIELD: 12 MUFFINS

1½ cups shredded zucchini (about 2 small zucchini)

2 cups whole-grain pancake or biscuit mix

1 teaspoon cinnamon

1 teaspoon allspice

2 eggs

¾ cup brown sugar

¼ cup unsweetened applesauce

2 teaspoons fresh lemon juice

Nonstick spray or paper liners

Powdered sugar (enough to dust the muffins)

Wash the zucchini and remove ends. Shred zucchini using largest holes on grater. Place the grated zucchini on paper towels and squeeze to remove water. Measure 1½ cups of squeezed-dry zucchini. Preheat the oven to 375°F. Line a twelve-cup muffin tin with paper liners or lightly spray with nonstick spray.

In a large bowl, mix whole-grain pancake mix (or biscuit mix) with spices. In a separate bowl, whisk together the eggs, brown sugar, applesauce, and lemon juice. Fold the egg-sugar mixture and shredded zucchini into the pancake-spice mixture; do not over mix.

Fill each muffin cup two-thirds full with batter. Bake 10 to 15 minutes or until golden. Remove muffins from tin and cool on a wire rack. Sprinkle muffins with a dusting of powdered sugar.

EYE-OPENING BREAKFAST BURRITOS

YIELD: 2 BURRITOS

2 whole-wheat tortillas

Nonstick cooking spray

1 red pepper, chopped

1 green pepper, chopped

1/2 onion, chopped

2 whole eggs and 4 egg whites, lightly beaten

1/2 teaspoon salt

1/4 teaspoon cayenne pepper

1/4 cup salsa

Preheat oven to 250°F. Place tortillas directly on rack in oven. Spray a frying pan with cooking spray. Sauté the peppers and onions over medium-low heat until tender. In a bowl, whisk together the eggs, salt, and cayenne pepper. Then add the egg mixture to the pan.

Cook until eggs reach desired consistency, stirring occasionally to keep eggs from sticking. Divide mixture onto warm tortillas, roll up tortillas, and top with salsa.

FABULOUS FRENCH TOAST

YIELD: 2 SLICES

1 egg

¼ cup skim or 1 percent milk

Dash of vanilla extract

2 slices of whole-wheat bread

Nonstick cooking spray

Cinnamon (optional)

Crack the egg into a medium-size bowl and beat well. Then mix in the milk and vanilla extract. Dunk each piece of bread in the egg mixture. Make sure the bread is totally covered. Let sit for several minutes until egg mixture is absorbed.

Spray a frying pan with cooking spray. Heat the pan on the stovetop over medium heat.

When the pan is warm, lower the heat. Add the bread and cook over low heat until the underside is light brown (about 5 minutes). Use a spatula to flip the bread over, and cook again for another 5 minutes. Transfer the French toast to a plate. Optional: Sprinkle powdered cinnamon for taste.

FRUIT SMOOTHIE

YIELD: 1 DRINK

Ice cubes

1 cup skim or 1 percent milk

⅓ cup low-fat cottage cheese

⅔ cup frozen strawberries or any other fruit of choice

1 teaspoon vanilla extract

Put all the ingredients into a blender. Put the lid on and blend for 45 to 60 seconds until smooth. Pour smoothie into a glass and enjoy.

LUNCH

Plan a healthy lunch. Review the school's lunch menu weekly and plan to have them bring a packed lunch on days they are not serving healthy options. You might send your kids with a lunch on days when they're serving pizza or fried chicken, and have them buy their lunch on days when they serve baked chicken and veggies. A well-packed lunch box should include:

- Turkey, chicken, ham, or tuna fish sandwich on whole-wheat bread
- Tons of uncooked vegetables (pick your child's favorites and they'll eat plenty of them)
- Fresh fruit
- Skim or 1 percent milk, or water

Below are some more recipes to offer your kids for a healthy lunch.

BITE-SIZE PIZZA

YIELD: 8 TO 12 MINI-SLICES

4 to 6 mini-wheat bagels, cut in half

Tomato sauce

Part-skim mozzarella cheese, shredded

Toppings like diced green pepper, chopped onion, or chopped tomato

12 slices mini, precooked Canadian bacon or ham

Seasonings like oregano, basil, and pepper

Preheat oven to 325 or 350°F. Spread tomato sauce on each bagel half. Sprinkle the shredded cheese all over the tomato sauce on each half. Distribute the Canadian bacon (or ham) equally. Add your favorite toppings. Put a light sprinkling of seasonings on each half.

Put the bagel halves on the baking sheet. Bake in the oven for about 5 to 8 minutes. You'll know they're done when the cheese is bubbly. Let cool for a minute, then enjoy these tiny pizzas!

GRILLED CHEESE

YIELD: 1 SANDWICH

1 ounce light cheddar cheese, sliced

2 slices whole-wheat bread

2 tablespoons egg whites or egg substitute

1 tablespoon skim or 1 percent milk

Nonstick cooking spray

Place cheese on one slice of bread. Top with remaining bread slice. In a shallow bowl, combine egg substitute and skim milk. Spray cooking spray in a large nonstick skillet. Dip sandwich in egg mixture and place in heated skillet. Cook sandwich over medium heat for 3 minutes on each side or until golden.

HANDY WRAPS

YIELD: 1 WRAP PER PERSON

1 package whole-wheat tortillas

Mustard and light mayonnaise

Lean cold cuts, sliced from the deli (ham and turkey)

Low-fat cheese slices

Chopped vegetables (your choice)

Lay a tortilla out flat and spread with mayonnaise and mustard. Then layer with a slice of ham and a slice of turkey. Next add a slice of cheese. Add vegetables. Roll up the wrap and cut into round bite-sized pieces. Pack in an airtight container. Simple to make and great for school lunches!

MEATBALL SUBS

YIELD: 1 SANDWICH (RECOMMENDED)

1 pound 93 percent extra-lean ground beef

$\frac{1}{2}$ cup whole-grain breadcrumbs

1 egg

1 teaspoon seasoned salt or herb seasoning mix

Nonstick cooking spray

1 cup meatless spaghetti sauce

Part-skim mozzarella cheese, grated

Whole-wheat hoagie buns

Mix together ground beef, breadcrumbs, egg, and seasoning. Shape into 1 $\frac{1}{2}$ inch-sized balls. Spray pan with cooking spray. Brown in skillet over medium heat. Add in spaghetti sauce and heat thoroughly. Spoon meatballs and sauce onto split rolls, sprinkle with cheese and serve. (Okay to make the night before for school lunch. Store in an airtight container in the refrigerator. Can be microwave heated at school.)

HEALTHY HOT DOGS

YIELD: 1 OR 2 HOT DOGS (RECOMMENDED)

Turkey or chicken hot dogs

Whole-grain buns

Mustard

Ketchup

Low-fat cheese

Warm turkey or chicken dogs, load in whole-grain buns, add your favorite healthy toppings.

SNACKING

Snacking is important to keep your kids' energy levels high throughout the day. But the snacks must be healthy snacks. Have these snacks ready for your kids to eat after school:

- Whole-wheat bread with peanut butter

- Whole-grain crackers, lean deli meats, and 2 percent cheese

- Fruit with low-fat cottage cheese

- Fruit with almonds or walnuts

- Fruit with string cheese

- Microwave popcorn

- Salsa with uncooked or lightly steamed vegetables

Here are some other healthy snacks you can offer your kids to boost their energy levels and help them control their weight.

FRUIT KABOBS

YIELD: 4 KABOBS

1 apple

1 banana

1/3 cup red seedless grapes

1/3 cup green seedless grapes

2/3 cup pineapple chunks

1 cup light yogurt

1/4 cup dried coconut, shredded

After washing the fruit, cut the apple and banana into small squares, and the grapes into halves. Put the fruit and yogurt each onto a large plate. Spread the shredded coconut onto another large plate.

Slide the pieces of fruit onto a skewer and design your own kabob by putting as much or as little of whatever fruit your child may want! Do this until the stick is almost covered from end to end. Hold the kabob at the ends and roll it in the yogurt, so the fruit gets covered. Then roll it in the coconut.

Repeat these steps with another skewer.

HEALTHY TRAIL MIX

YIELD: 3 CUPS

1 cup whole-grain cereal

1 cup dried fruit of your choice

1 cup nuts such as walnut pieces, slivered almonds, or pistachios

Cinnamon to taste

Measure out ingredients. Combine in large bowl. Use single-serving bags or containers to take this snack on the go.

SOUR APPLE SLICES

YIELD: 2 CUPS

3 Granny Smith apples

Lemon juice

Cut the apples into thin slices and place them in a large freezer bag. With the bag upright, squeeze the juice from the lemon over the cut apples. Seal bag and place in the fridge to enjoy cold!

AWESOME APPLESAUCE

YIELD: 2 SERVINGS

2 small red apples, peeled

2 tablespoons lemon juice

2 pinches of cinnamon

Peel the apples and cut them into small pieces. Throw out the cores. Put the apple pieces and lemon juice into a blender or food processor. Blend until the mixture is very smooth. Pour the mixture into two small bowls and stir in the cinnamon. Enjoy your awesome applesauce!

HUMMUS

YIELD: 2 CUPS

15-ounce can garbanzo beans, drained
(set the liquid aside)

2 garlic cloves, minced

1 teaspoon ground cumin

1 tablespoon olive oil

Salt and freshly ground pepper to taste

Combine the garbanzo beans, garlic, cumin, and olive oil in a food processor. Blend on low speed, gradually adding reserved garbanzo bean liquid, until desired consistency is achieved. Add salt and pepper to taste. Use uncooked or lightly steamed vegetables, whole-wheat crackers, or pita bread for dipping.

DINNER

Supper is usually our largest meal. However, if we eat right all day long, it should be our smallest meal. Pay close attention to how much you are putting on your child's plate; only put what you know they can comfortably eat. Generally, dinners should include:

- Baked or broiled lean animal protein (chicken, fish, sirloin, center-cut pork chop, and lean or extra-lean ground beef)
- Vegetables, cooked or in a salad
- Healthy unsaturated fats (olive oil, nuts/seeds, avocado)
- Healthy carbohydrates (whole-wheat pasta/bread, brown rice, fruit, etc.)

More healthy supper recipes follow.

VEGETABLE LASAGNA

YIELD: 6–8 SERVINGS

1 pound zucchini

1 pound summer squash

1/4 teaspoon Italian seasoning

1/4 teaspoon freshly ground pepper

2 cups tomato pasta sauce

3 cups fresh spinach, trimmed and chopped

16 ounces low-fat cottage cheese

1 cup fresh basil leaves

2 egg yolks

1/3 cup Parmesan cheese

2/3 cup seasoned whole-grain breadcrumbs

2 cups part-skim mozzarella, shredded

Nonstick cooking spray

Heat oven to 425°F. Coat two large baking pans with nonstick cooking spray. Cut the squash and zucchini lengthwise in half. Then, cut each half lengthwise into slices about 1/4 inch thick. Spread the squash and zucchini slices on the pans in single layer and season with Italian seasoning and pepper. Bake for 25 minutes, turning over once halfway through baking. Remove from the oven and set aside. Reduce oven temperature to 375°F.

In a large skillet, heat pasta sauce over medium-high heat. Mix chopped spinach into the pasta sauce. Stir frequently and heat until warm and spinach is reduced.

In a food processor, combine the cottage cheese, basil, egg yolks, and 2 tablespoons of the Parmesan cheese. Blend until all ingredients are combined and smooth.

To assemble, sprinkle 2 tablespoons of breadcrumbs over the bottom of a 13- x 9- x 2-inch baking pan. Cover the bottom of the dish with half of the zucchini and squash slices. Next, spread the cottage cheese mixture over the squash and zucchini slices. Sprinkle with 3 tablespoons of breadcrumbs. Top with remaining zucchini and squash slices. Sprinkle with the remaining 3 tablespoons of breadcrumbs. Pour pasta sauce evenly over the top. Sprinkle mozzarella cheese evenly over the top. Sprinkle with the remaining Parmesan cheese.

Bake for approximately 35 minutes. Cheese should be browned and bubbling. Let stand for 10 to 15 minutes before serving.

Variation: Try adding 93 percent extra-lean ground beef. Brown first, then add to warmed pasta sauce.

CONFETTI RICE

YIELD: 7 CUPS

1 tablespoon olive oil

½ cup asparagus, finely chopped

½ cup scallions, finely chopped

½ cup celery, finely chopped

1 cup fresh spinach, chopped

1 medium carrot, grated (approximately 1 cup)

3 cloves garlic, finely chopped

Juice of one lemon

2 tablespoons soy sauce

¼ teaspoon freshly ground pepper

4 cups cooked brown rice

In a large skillet, heat the oil over medium heat until hot. Carefully add the asparagus, scallions, celery, spinach, and carrots. Stir quickly for 2 minutes. Then add the garlic, lemon juice, soy sauce, and pepper. Continue stirring for 1 minute. Add the cooked rice, mixing well until heated through. Serve immediately.

Variation: Two cups of cooked, diced chicken or turkey sausage can be added to make this an easy one-pan main dish. Add to skillet after stir-frying vegetables and before adding the seasonings.

HOMESTYLE "FRIED" CHICKEN

YIELD: 4 SERVINGS

1/4 cup breadcrumbs (preferably whole wheat)

1 tablespoon grated Parmesan cheese

1 teaspoon paprika

1 teaspoon dried thyme

1/2 teaspoon garlic salt

1/4 teaspoon cayenne pepper

1/3 cup low-fat buttermilk

4 skinless chicken breasts (6 ounces each)

Nonstick cooking spray

1 tablespoon butter, melted

Preheat oven to 400°F. Combine the breadcrumbs, Parmesan, paprika, thyme, garlic salt, and cayenne pepper in a shallow dish. Pour buttermilk into a separate shallow dish.

Dip chicken in buttermilk, then dredge in breadcrumb mixture. Place in baking pan coated with cooking spray and drizzle butter over chicken. Bake 40 minutes or until done.

ORIENTAL-STYLE PORK CHOPS

YIELD: 4 SERVINGS

4 center-cut pork chops (thin cut, 6 ounces each)

2 tablespoons sesame oil

1 medium onion, cut into 1/2-inch pieces

3 carrots, peeled and thinly sliced

10 fresh mushrooms, cut into 1/4-inch pieces

2 cups broccoli florets

4 tablespoons low-sodium soy sauce

5 baby corns, canned

Freshly ground pepper to taste

In a medium-size frying pan, sauté pork chops in sesame oil for 2 minutes on each side. Remove from pan and set aside.

To the same pan, add onions, carrots, and mushrooms, and sauté until tender. Add broccoli and soy sauce and cook 3 minutes. Add the baby corn and cook 1 minute. Return pork chops to pan. Add pepper to taste.

Buffalo "Wings" with Blue Cheese Dip

YIELD: 12 SERVINGS

Nonstick cooking spray

12 skinless chicken tenders

1 1/4 ounce taco seasoning packet

1/2 cup light sour cream

2 tablespoons crumbled blue cheese

2 tablespoons skim or 1 percent milk

4 medium celery stalks, cut into 2-inch pieces

Preheat the oven to 400°F. Coat a large baking sheet with cooking spray. Put chicken tenders in a plastic bag. Add taco seasoning. Seal bag and shake to coat. Place chicken on baking sheet. Bake for approximately 18 to 20 minutes (times will vary) until cooked through.

Stir together sour cream, blue cheese, and milk for the dip. Serve chicken with dip and celery on the side.

Variation: Shrimp or crawfish (shells removed and cleaned) may be substituted for the chicken tenders.

CHEESY MAC & CHEESE

YIELD: 12 SERVINGS

Nonstick cooking spray

2 teaspoons whole-wheat flour

1 1/3 cups skim or 1 percent milk

1 cup shredded low-fat sharp cheddar cheese

1 cup shredded part-skim mozzarella cheese, divided

1/2 teaspoon salt

6 cups cooked whole-wheat penne or macaroni

Preheat the oven to 400°F. Spray a casserole dish with cooking spray. In a medium-sized bowl, mix flour with 1/4 cup milk, forming a paste. Pour mixture into a medium saucepan, and stir in remainder of milk. Add all the cheddar cheese, half of the mozzarella cheese, and salt. Cook over medium heat, stirring until cheese melts and mixture thickens. When mixture is smooth and thickened, remove from heat.

In a large bowl, pour cheese mixture over cooked macaroni or penne, stirring well. Transfer the macaroni and cheese to the casserole dish, sprinkling remaining mozzarella over the top. Bake for 20 to 25 minutes until heated through and lightly browned.

Variation: Cooked diced chicken or 93 percent extra-lean ground beef can be added to make this an easy one-pan main dish. Add to cooked macaroni or penne after stirring in cheese mixture.

HEARTY HOMEMADE CHILI

YIELD: 12 SERVINGS

1 tablespoon olive oil

1 cup chopped green peppers

1 cup chopped onions

1 tablespoon minced garlic

2 tablespoons chili powder

1 pound ground turkey breast

16 ounces salsa

3 cups canned, fat-free, reduced-sodium chicken broth

30-ounces canned kidney beans, rinsed and drained

1 tablespoon tomato paste

Salt and pepper to taste

$\frac{1}{2}$ cup each of light sour cream, chopped tomato, low-fat shredded cheddar cheese for garnish

Heat oil in large saucepan over medium heat. Add peppers, onions, and garlic. Cook until onions are golden brown. Stir in chili powder and cook 1 to 2 more minutes. Add ground turkey, stirring well. Cook 5 to 6 minutes or until meat is browned. Transfer mixture to a large, deep pot.

Add salsa, chicken broth, beans, and tomato paste. Bring to a simmer over medium heat. Reduce heat and simmer until chili has thickened (approximately 45 minutes). Add salt and pepper to taste. Serve with dollop of sour cream, chopped tomato, and cheddar cheese.

MEATLOAF

YIELD: 12 SERVINGS

Nonstick cooking spray

2 pounds extra-lean ground beef

$1/2$ cup ground flaxseed

$1/4$ cup whole-wheat breadcrumbs

2 egg whites, lightly beaten

$1/4$ teaspoon chopped garlic

2 teaspoons Dijon mustard

3 tablespoons Parmesan cheese

1 cup chopped mushrooms

1 cup fresh chopped spinach

$1/2$ cup marinara sauce

$1/2$ cup canned, fat-free, reduced-sodium
chicken broth

Freshly ground pepper to taste

Ketchup to taste

Preheat the oven to 350°F. Spray two loaf pans with cooking spray. In a large bowl, mix all the ingredients except ketchup together thoroughly. Divide mixture into loaf pans and top with ketchup. Bake 30 to 35 minutes, until the top is golden and rounded. Take care not to overcook. The loaf should be firm when you give the pan a shake.

CAJUN JAMBALAYA

YIELD: 6–8 SERVINGS

1 tablespoon canola oil

10 ounces soy or turkey sausage links
sliced into 1-inch pieces

2 cups chopped onions

1 cup chopped celery

1 cup chopped green pepper

3 small bay leaves

4 tablespoons minced garlic

2 tablespoons Cajun seasoning

$\frac{1}{2}$ teaspoon salt

2 cups brown rice

3 cups tomato juice

3 cups canned, fat-free, reduced-sodium chicken broth

1 pound fresh chopped tomatoes
or 14-ounce can chopped tomatoes

In a large pot, heat oil over medium-high heat. Sauté sausage links for 15 minutes or until browned. Add the onions, celery, green pepper, bay leaves, garlic, Cajun seasoning, and salt. Continue to cook for 10 to 12 minutes, stirring frequently, until the onions are browned. Stir in rice and cook 5 more minutes, stirring occasionally. Add tomato juice and chicken broth, stirring well, and bring to a boil. Reduce heat to medium and simmer, covered, for 15 minutes. Add tomatoes, stirring well. Continue cooking over low heat, covered, until rice is tender (about 1 hour).

WHAT PARENTS CAN DO

In order for this healthy eating plan to be a lifestyle and not a temporary "diet," children must have variety in their food choices. Allowing them to select new, healthy recipes and to help with the preparation of food teaches them not only what types of food are good for them, but it also encourages them to try new foods. It is well known that children who help cook and prepare their own foods are more likely to eat those foods.

The recipes presented in this chapter are just a few meal suggestions among the many options available. For additional healthy recipes aimed at helping your child maintain a healthy weight, I encourage you to consult other sources available in bookstores, libraries, and on the Internet.

CHAPTER 6 SUMMARY

- Eating right is one of the keys to an effective fat-loss plan for kids.

- Healthy breakfast, lunch, dinner, and snacks are encouraged to help maintain satiety, prevent hunger, and prevent overeating or bingeing.

- With little extra thought and preparation these meals can be fun, healthy, and quick to put together.

PART FOUR

The Fitness Plan for Kids and Parents

CHAPTER 7

Staying Active to Stay Lean

The Benefits of Getting Your Child Moving

Being active is vitally important for children. Not only does it enhance their physical and mental health during their formative years, but it can also help them establish patterns that can be beneficial to them as they grow into adulthood.

Until recently childhood and adolescence were times of significant physical activity, relatively free of serious health problems (not counting injuries that may have resulted from these activities). However, sports and exercise have become less and less a part of our kids' lives in our high-tech age. The proliferation of and easy access to computers, video games, iPods, cable television, cell phones, and other sedentary diversions has made it possible for kids to experience adventures without physical activity. Not only do sedentary children lose out on the obvious health benefits of activity, but their communications skills, goal-setting abilities, and general attitudes are sacrificed as well.

In a report that researchers termed "the first of its kind," the National Institutes of Health (NIH) and Common Sense Media, a nonprofit advocacy group, studied the effects of media consumption on the health of young people. The group's findings were reported in an article in *The New York Times*, dated December 1, 2008. According to the article, the report concluded that "a strong correlation exists between greater exposure [to electronic media] and adverse health outcomes."

Among those "adverse health outcomes" cited were a rise in childhood obesity, along with increased usage of alcohol, tobacco, and drugs, and low academic achievement.

The report was the result of a review of 173 separate studies undertaken since 1980 relating to how media consumption affects children's health. One of the five members of the review panel was Dr. Ezekiel J. Emmanuel, chairman of the NIH's bioethics department and brother of President Barack Obama's chief of staff, Rahm Emmanuel, and because of that connection, the problem is expected to get some attention during the Obama administration. During his campaign for the presidency, Obama, a former college athlete, repeatedly urged parents to "turn off the television set and put the video games away" in his speeches and commercials.

In years' past, a child could get his or her exercise in school. Today, an alarming 75 percent of physical education classes nationwide have become casualties of budget cuts and an unfortunate prevailing attitude that PE is a non-essential part of the academic curriculum. Very few states at the present time require PE and, sadly, some of the consequences of that are beginning to show. (See Appendix B for the physical education requirements for your state.)

FITNESS MATTERS: THE BOGALUSA HEART STUDY

The most powerful argument for rethinking the American child's exercise, diet, and lifestyle habits comes from the famous, decades-old Bogalusa Heart Study. The study, the longest and most detailed study of cardiovascular risk factors in children in the world, tracked the health and lifestyle habits of more than 16,000 people from childhood to adulthood for thirty-three years. The federally funded study has shown that the seeds of heart disease begin germinating early in life and are directly related to obesity and lack of exercise. The study, which has held up as a measuring stick for young people in other communities around the country, has also been held up an omen for the future if the trends toward childhood obesity aren't reversed soon.

For their working model, researchers, led by Gerald S. Berenson, MD, director of the Tulane Center for Cardiovascular Health, chose the small, rural, racially mixed city of Bogalusa, Louisiana, and its surrounding area in Washington Parish (county). The study brought together a multidisciplinary team of anthropologists, biochemists, cardiologists, epidemiologists, geneticists, nurses, nutritionists, psychologists, sociologists, and statisticians, who worked jointly to study hereditary and environmental aspects of early coronary artery disease and hypertension.

From 1972 to 2005, the group tracked 16,000 Black-American and Caucasian children and young adults, many of them since birth, with annual physical examinations that included a blood test for cholesterol and other harmful blood fats and blood pressure measurement. Details on their height, weight, dietary habits, tobacco use, and physical activity were recorded. The investigators found that children as young as two were consuming a high-fat, high-sodium, low-fiber diet that, unfortunately, has become fairly typical among American children. The study group covered a broad spectrum of individuals and individual activity levels, ranging from those who were largely inactive to those who were healthy, athletic, and active.

One of the most startling conclusions of the Bogalusa Heart Study, was that heart disease can begin developing much earlier than had been previously thought possible. Autopsy studies of American soldiers who died in the Korean War (1950–1953) had already demonstrated that heart disease can begin as early as age eighteen, but the Bogalusa Study produced pathological evidence that these conditions can actually start sooner. Grossly visible fatty streaks were seen in the aortas of some of the children studied after age three and were found in the coronary arteries beginning in the second decade of life, nearly twenty years after the study began.

The study also conducted autopsies on 204 participants, aged two to thirty-nine years, who died during the study period. The autopsy results, published by Dr. Berenson and his colleagues in the *New England Journal of Medicine* (June 4, 1998), found that all participants had fatty streaks in the aorta, and that the prevalence of fatty streaks in the coronary arteries increased with age. Both conditions are associated with several known risk factors for heart disease, including high blood pressure, smoking, obesity, and elevated levels of very low-density lipoprotein (VLDL) cholesterol— the worst kind of bad cholesterol. The higher the number of risk factors, the greater the extent of fatty streak lesions, the study findings pointed out. In short, the predictors of heart disease in children are similar to those in middle-aged people. Heart disease prevention, therefore, should start early in life, the authors of the article concluded.

Dr. Berenson was quoted in the article as advising a reduction in the amount of saturated fat and cholesterol in a child's diet. Dr. Berenson said that the study's results are representative of what is happening to children across the nation: "They're getting heavier, not taller." The study was also able to draw conclusions based on race and gender, citing proclivities of Black-American and Caucasian males and females toward specific ailments or physical conditions. It has been cited as a model upon which many conclusions about childhood obesity can be drawn.

Aftermath of the Study and Its Impact

The findings brought out by the Bogalusa Heart Study have been corroborated by other studies over the years. A study conducted by University of South Carolina exercise-scientist Russell R. Pate, PhD, and colleagues concluded that one in three (33 percent) of teenaged boys and girls fail to meet acceptable fitness standards. Their finding, which was reported in the *Archives of Pediatrics* (October 2006), was based on a national sample of 3,287 kids between the ages of twelve and nineteen.

The study measured the youths' heart rates and oxygen intake during short treadmill tests. Even more shocking was the finding that the least-fit age group among those tested was the twelve- to thirteen-year-olds. Almost 45 percent, nearly half of the kids in this age group, failed to meet fitness standards. Not surprising was the fact that the least-fit kids among those tested were those who were overweight and less active than their peers. These tendencies may very well have developed when these kids were younger and got worse as they got older.

I could go on and on, citing study after study, linking the likelihood of childhood obesity to medical problems experienced in later adulthood but I think the point has been made. We need to get a handle on the problem of childhood obesity and reverse it before it's too late. It is already a national epidemic that could become endemic in the next generation.

ESTABLISHING A DAILY FITNESS ROUTINE

The next best thing—after developing good eating habits—is a program of moderate to vigorous exercise. The metabolism of an overweight, sedentary child is sluggish and inefficient at utilizing calories. Activity and exercise are the keys to stimulating a child's metabolism to burn fat. A growing child's metabolism is much more active than an adult's. Think of it as a small, powerful furnace. But this furnace must be "stoked" properly to reach maximum efficiency. When metabolism is stimulated properly through higher levels of activity—and fueled correctly through healthier nutritional habits—children naturally begin to lose weight as they grow.

Regular exercise improves a child's ratio of good to bad cholesterol (lipid profile), reduces blood pressure, increases elasticity in the major arteries, and helps to balance the body's hormonal systems. Research also has shown that exercise helps kids deal better with stress and it improves mood, making kids generally happier and more emotionally balanced. Children who are active not only become leaner, but also their levels of self-esteem and confidence are significantly higher compared to children who are sedentary. They also generally perform better in school, as attested to by numerous studies.

The American Heart Association (AHA) recommends at least sixty minutes of moderate to vigorous physical activity daily for kids. I concur with this recommendation, although, for kids who have been engaging in little or no physical activity, it is best if they start out in smaller increments and gradually work up to sixty minutes or more. They should start out with fifteen to twenty minutes of exercise or other physical activity, continue that for a few weeks, then work up to thirty minutes, then forty-five, then sixty. This is a good way to get them into the exercise/activity habit without forcing too much on them at once.

Pediatric endocrinologist Robert Gensure (mentioned in Chapter 2) suggests that overweight or otherwise inactive children begin by walking half a mile to a mile each day outdoors or at home on a treadmill. He recommends that they use a pedometer to help them keep track of these small daily step goals and as they work their way up from there.

In a landmark paper on childhood obesity published by Colorado

State University Extension in the late 1990s, nutrition specialists Patricia Kendall, Karen Wilken and Elena Serrano highlight three important concepts needed to enhance the impact of physical activity on health, as well as the child's interest in it. These are as follows:

- **Time:** Children should take part in at least sixty minutes of age and developmentally appropriate activities every day.

- **Intensity:** Activity periods should last ten to fifteen minutes or more and include a range of intensities (moderate to vigorous).

- **Variety:** Children should engage in a variety of physical activities of various levels of intensity.

At about the same time, the Centers for Disease Control (CDC) recommended that schools establish policies that promote enjoyable, lifelong physical activity among young people. Their guidelines stated, "Physical education should emphasize skills for lifetime physical activities (for example, dance, strength training, jogging, swimming, bicycling, cross-country skiing, walking, and hiking) rather than those for competitive sports." These guidelines also recommend that fitness-enhancing physical activities become an integral part of the American family's lifestyle.

Ten years after publication of the paper, many of these same concepts and recommendations were included in the report by the Expert Committee on the Assessment, Prevention and Treatment of Child and Adolescent Overweight and Obesity, which would tend to indicate that the problem has not gotten better. (See Appendix A for a copy of the report.) In fact, it may have gotten worse. Technology over the past decade has advanced so much that today's children have even more passive devices at their disposal to lead them into a more sedentary lifestyle. This is where parental involvement and intervention come in.

WHAT PARENTS CAN DO

For best success, all family members should set good examples and should participate in this increased physical activity. If parents want to help their

TEN IDEAS TO GET ACTIVE

Don't just sit there, get up and moving! It's easy—and fun—to work in a little extra activity. Here are ten ideas to get you and your kids moving from the President's Challenge Physical Activity and Fitness Awards Program.

Kids

1. Take your dog out for a walk.
2. Start up a playground kickball game.
3. Join a sports team.
4. Go to the park with a friend.
5. Help your parents with yardwork.
6. Play tag with kids in your neighborhood.
7. Ride your bike to school.
8. Walk to the store for your mom.
9. See how many jumping jacks you can do.
10. Race a friend to the end of the block.

Adults

1. Use a push mower to mow the lawn.
2. Go for a walk in a nearby park.
3. Take the stairs instead of an elevator.
4. Bike to work, to run errands, or visit friends.
5. Clean out the garage or the attic.
6. Walk with a friend over the lunch hour.
7. Volunteer to become a coach or referee.
8. Sign up for an group exercise class.
9. Join a softball league.
10. Park at the farthest end of the lot.

overweight or obese child attain a healthier weight, they must stop being couch potatoes themselves. They not only have to set a good example for their kids, they have to stop letting the TV sets and computers babysit their kids as well. They have to take control of the amount of time their kids spend watching TV or playing video or computer games. They have to regulate the amount of time their kids spend text messaging and talking on the phone, especially cell phones.

But even these steps are not enough. To the extent they are physically able to do so, parents should provide good company for their children on bike rides, walks, swims, or other physical activities. They can play pitch and catch with their kids, toss the football back and forth, shoot baskets together with portable hoops, or take them out to the nearest public tennis court. Physical activity should be fun and should make children feel good, not a chore they must do to lose weight.

A recent paper published by the National Institute of Diabetes & Digestive & Kidney Diseases: Weight-control Information Network (WIN) details a number of things parents can do to help and encourage their children to lose weight. It advises: "One of the most important things you can do to help overweight children is to let them know that they are okay, whatever their weight. Children's feelings about themselves often are based on their parents' feelings about them. If you accept your children at any weight, they will be more likely to accept and feel good about themselves. It is also important to talk to your children about weight, allowing them to share their concerns with you. You child probably knows better than anyone else that he or she has a weight problem. For this reason, overweight children need support, acceptance, and encouragement from their parents."

The WIN paper also urges parents not to single out their overweight child if they have other children who are of a normal weight for their size and age group. They also urge parents to increase their levels of activity, as well as those of their children. Some of their suggestions are as follows:

• Be a role model for your children. If you want physically active kids, be active yourself. If your children see that you are active and having fun, they are likely to be active and stay active the rest of their lives.

- Plan family activities that provide everyone with exercise and enjoyment, like walking, dancing, biking or swimming. Go walking or bike riding after dinner instead of watching TV. Make sure that you plan activities that are in a safe environment.

- Be sensitive to your child's needs. Overweight children may feel uncomfortable about participating in certain activities. It is important to help your child find physical activities that they enjoy and that aren't embarrassing or too difficult. Brainstorm with them about a variety of activities that may be a good match for their personality, ability, and age. Then let your child choose the activities that feel right to them

- Reduce the amount of time you and your family spend in sedentary activities, such as watching TV or playing video games. Keep these activities to no more than two hours daily.

- Become more active throughout the day and encourage your family to do so as well. For example, walk up the stairs instead of taking the elevator, or do some activity during a work or school break. Get up and stretch or just walk around.

- Put it on paper. A written plan can encourage your child to stay on track. Chapter 10 contains an Exercise Diary you can use as a model.

The point is not to make physical activity an unwelcome chore. That could have the opposite effect and turn your child off about losing weight and staying in shape. Don't be overbearing or demanding on your child. Don't do or say anything that could make them feel inferior because of their weight or physical condition. That, too, could scar them for life and make them resentful of any activity that requires even the slightest bit of exertion.

There are many activities parents and kids can do together that can keep the mind and body sharp yet don't require a lot of exertion and effort. In Chapter 9, I will share some of them. Playtime is important, too, as I will discuss next.

CHAPTER 7 SUMMARY

- It is vitally important for children to be physically active not only to enhance their physical and mental health during their formative years, but also to establish patterns that can benefit them in the future.

- Exercise has many benefits, including increased metabolic rates, improved ratio of good to bad cholesterol, reduced blood pressure, greater stress relief, and increased self-esteem.

- If exercise is not currently a part of the child's daily routine, start off slow and build up to an established goal in the form of time commitment and activity choice, while setting daily step goals with use of a pedometer.

- All family members must set good examples and should participate in this increased physical activity with their children.

- Do not make exercise a physical chore. Allow children to participate in activities that are fun and enjoyable to them as individuals.

CHAPTER 8

Creative Play

The Importance of Encouraging Activity for Your Child

As we continue to examine the problems of overweight and obesity in children today and try to devise solutions, I don't want to overlook one of the most important components of a child's growing-up process: what they do during their playtime.

By "playtime" I'm not necessarily talking about their participation in competitive sports, although this, too, is an important aspect of their physical and mental development. Playtime can involve not only physical activities, but also those that challenge their social skills. The formative years between eight and twelve are a crucial time in which their personalities, as well as their bodies, are developing traits that can very well last them into adolescence and adulthood. Therefore, the interactive pastimes they engage in at these ages (as long as they're not destructive) should be encouraged by parents—not discouraged.

Education has always been a key factor in the forward progress of this country, as it has been in all cultures since civilization began. Only a well-educated populace can sustain the framework of an orderly society in which we can make free choices of leadership and vocations. Only a well-educated, enlightened populace can keep us from descending into a dark age in which people are left to fend for themselves and become susceptible to diseases, superstitions, and the predations of other, more warlike and aggressive members of our human species. Making sure that our children are well-educated helps prepare them for the challenges they will face later in life. Also, it ensures us that the level of civilization we have thus far attained will continue and hopefully improve into our children's generation and the generations beyond that.

However, "book learning," as some might call it, is only one component of a child's growing-up process. As important as it is for children to learn math, science, the arts, language skills, and the history of our nation and other cultures, it is equally important for them to learn interactive skills. These interactive skills involve how they relate to other children, as well as to the adults around them. They are not necessarily skills the schools can teach them in the classroom, but, in many cases, they are skills the schools can encourage them to learn.

TAKING PLAY SERIOUSLY

An enlightening article on the importance of play, titled "Taking Play Seriously," appeared in a recent issue of the *New York Times Magazine* (February 17, 2008). In it, reporter Robin Marantz Henig cites a number of recent studies and experts in early childhood development, who insist that play is extremely beneficial for growing children.

The article is one of the most insightful articles I've read in a long time, and it confirmed much of what I have been advocating for many years. I do a lot of reading with subscriptions to a dozen or more journals, some of which are of a scholarly bent, but this article resonated with me in such a profound way that I decided to make the topic the primary focus of this chapter. During my thirty-plus years of working as a performance enhancement specialist, I've always felt that playtime is an important component of a child's growing-up process. Among other things, it can help reinforce healthy eating and exercise habits.

The article extensively quotes Stuart Brown, MD, president of the National Institute for Play and a highly respected authority on the subject. He founded the institute in 1996 after twenty years of psychiatric practice and research convinced him of the potentially harmful long-term consequences of play deprivation. During a talk before a capacity crowd at the New York Public Library in January 2008, Dr. Brown called play part of the "developmental sequencing of becoming a human primate. If you look at what produces learning and memory and well-being, play is as fundamental as any other aspect of life, including sleep and dreams."

In his talks and in other seminars and forums, including a radio show he co-hosts, Dr. Brown touches a sensitive nerve among the various audiences at which his message is aimed. Educators are concerned that their higher-ups in school hierarchies are cutting down on kids' recess and increasing teaching demands on their already crammed curriculum. Psychologists complain that the loss of kids' creative and often unstructured playtime is depriving them of a vital component of their normal growing-up processes. Parents, themselves, even bemoan the fact that their kids don't play as they did when they were kids—their offspring often opting for more passive pursuits like TV watching, and computer and video games. And, perhaps most importantly, as far as the aim of this book and my Body Plan for Kids program is concerned, insufficient playtime may be linked to the alarming rise in childhood obesity.

The article clearly points out the dilemma parents face between allowing their kids to be kids and a compulsion to channel them toward goals that will benefit them in adulthood. It is a well-known fact that American students have been lagging behind other industrialized countries in the development of certain vital skills necessary to function in a technological age, particularly in math and science. Parents may feel compelled to push their kids into music or dance lessons or test-prep classes instead of letting them "do their thing" and enjoy their youth, playing by their own rules with their peers. Increased competition for a limited number of admissions slots in prestigious colleges and universities also has many parents concerned that their kids' free time could be better spent studying instead of playing.

Consequently, the discussion over the importance of play in kids' lives has risen above the level of being considered "frivolous," and has evolved into serious scientific and sociological study and laboratory testing. By studying play behaviors in animals—both in the wild and in controlled laboratory settings—scientists and other researchers make some very convincing arguments for the necessity of play in children. In their studies of animal play behaviors, they have come to some conclusions that may be equally applicable to humans.

THE BENEFITS OF PLAY

According to the *Times* article, "Scientists who study play, in animals and humans alike, are developing a consensus view that play is something more than a way for restless kids to work off steam, more than a way for chubby kids to burn off calories, more than a frivolous luxury. Play, in their view, is a central part of neurological growth and development—one important way that children build complex, skilled, responsive, socially adept and cognitively flexible brains."

Scientists who study evolutionary biology are quick to note that play is a component of nearly all mammals' early stages of life. Most species have anywhere from ten to one hundred distinct signals that they use to solicit play or reassure their "opponents" in play fighting that they are only playing and not being serious. Puppies and kittens, when wrestling with each other, are careful not to hurt each other. They generally hold back the full force of their playful scratching or biting yet, at the same time, they may be learning and practicing defensive moves that will ensure their survival when they become adults. "Through play, these movements can be learned when the stakes are low and then retrieved in adulthood, when the setting is less safe and the need for urgent," the article states. Likewise for children who when play fighting also tend to hold back and not hurt their playmates.

The article asserts that "an essential component of play is its frivolity," and quotes biologists who define play as "apparently purposeless activity." One authority who is quoted, Gordon Burghardt, PhD, wrote in his book *The Genesis of Animal Play* (MIT Press, 2005) that play is an activity of "limited immediate function." Nonetheless, Dr. Burghardt goes on to cite its necessity. Paraphrasing his theories, the reporter writes, "Play is an activity that is different from the non-play version of that activity (in terms of form, sequence, or the stage of life in which it occurs) . . . [it] is something the animal engages in voluntarily and repeatedly and occurs in a setting in which the animal is adequately fed, healthy, and free from stress."

That last part of Dr. Burghardt's definition would appear to imply that play is "the biological equivalent of a luxury item, the first thing to go when an animal or child is hungry or sick." Indeed, studies in the wild appear to back this contention. Monkeys, among the most notoriously playful mammals, will generally not play if food and/or water supplies are low or unavailable in their habitat. However, with human children, the equation can be more complicated. Being more complex than other mammals, human children will sometimes play even in the most depressing and deprived circumstances and environments. Sociologist George Eisen, in *Children and Play in the Holocaust* (University of Massachusetts Press, 1990) wrote, "Children's yearning for play naturally bursts forth, even amidst the horror."

However, according to the *Times* article, studies have shown that play levels diminish "when children suffer long-term, chronic deprivation, either one at a time in abusive or neglectful homes, or on a massive scale in times of famine, war, or forced relocation. And children can survive, albeit imperfectly, without it." Situations like these, in which children are deprived of play due to circumstances beyond their control, forces them to grow up in a hurry. Oftentimes they mature into adults, who are serious, humorless, and intensively focused on their sense of purpose. They may not be getting much enjoyment out of life beyond the satisfaction that comes with success in their chosen profession or vocation. Family and social life, and consequently, opportunities for career advancement may all suffer when an individual who had an unhappy childhood carries that unhappiness into adulthood.

In controlled-laboratory settings, biologists believe that the behavioral patterns they track in animals like rats, mice, and monkeys can be just as easily applied to humans. The reasons why this appears to be so became more clear the more the researchers studied the brains of their laboratory specimens and noted similarities in developmental patterns. Juvenile laboratory rats that were caged with other juvenile rats with whom they could play appeared to have more highly developed brains than those rats caged with adults that wouldn't play with them. Rats, like other mammals, are born with an overabundance of certain types of brain cells. As the animal matures, feedback that it receives and retains from the environment results in the selective elimination of excess brain cells. Play is believed to be one of the environmental factors that help in this pruning process of no-longer-necessary brain cells, whereas play deprivation interferes with that process.

This, the study conductors and other experts have theorized, could be analogous to humans. We're all familiar with the old cliché: "All work and no play makes Johnny a dull boy." Well, it now seems that studies are arriving at the same conclusion. Children raised with little or no play could have less developed brains than those who had adequate playtimes. These findings, they confidently feel, could provide a link to the still as yet unknown causes of attention deficit hyperactivity disorder (ADHD) in young children. It would be considered a major breakthrough if some-how, through all this research on play, a serious childhood disorder could be cured or at least better controlled. This, in turn, could help these children develop healthier eating patterns and exercise routines.

OTHER BENEFITS OF PLAY

Play appears to have other benefits as well. Marc Bekoff, PhD, an evolutionary biologist at the University of Colorado, calls play "a behavioral kaleidoscope" and "training for the unexpected." He believes it helps sharpen the senses in a way that helps the animal (and, by extension, humans) achieve success in group dominance, mate selection, avoiding capture, and locating food supplies. Other experts point to child studies that appear to show that those who engage in vigorous play activities tend to be more successful in their later adult endeavors. "Pretend play," for children around the age of four, may occupy about 20 percent of the child's day and, according to the article, "It includes some of the most wondrous moments of childhood: dramatic play, wordplay, ritual play, symbolic play, games, jokes, and imaginary friends."

Admittedly, play can get a bit rough for kids at times, especially when kids with bullying tendencies begin to dominate the weaker ones. This is usually the time when parents and/or teachers should assess the situation and its potential dangers and intervene when necessary. However, even situations like these are not all bad, according to some experts.

Brian Sutton-Smith, PhD, a psychologist who has taught at Columbia Teachers College and the University of Pennsylvania, in *The Ambigu-*

ity of Play (Harvard University Press, 2001), notes that in instances of rough play, children learn important life lessons that will help them in adulthood, even though those lessons may be unpleasant ones. "Children learn all those necessary arts of trickery, deception, harassment, divination, and foul play that their teachers won't teach them but are most important in successful human relationships in marriage, business, and war."

"In the end," the article concludes, "it comes down to a matter of trade-offs. There are only six hours in a school day, only another six or so till bedtime. Adults are forever trying to cram those hours with activities that are productive, educational, and (almost as an afterthought) fun. Animal findings about how play influences brain growth suggest that playing, though it might look silly and purposeless, warrants a place in every child's day. Not too overblown a place, not too sanctimonious a place, but a place that embraces all styles of play as every bit as essential to healthful neurological development as test-taking drills, Spanish lessons or Suzuki violin."

Which is pretty much how I would conclude the discussion on this topic as well.

WHAT PARENTS CAN DO

I advise all parents to let their kids be kids. As you would monitor what they eat, and how much TV they watch, computer time they log, and exercise they get, you should also allow ample playtime. As you have seen, play has benefits that contribute to your child's well-being. It can also foster a frame of mind in which they are more open and receptive to exercising and eating right. It's part of the overall package that can put them on the road to good health and keep them there.

CHAPTER 8 SUMMARY

- Let kids be kids. Playtime is beneficial for growing children.

- It is important to find a balance between work and play for children to put them on the road to good health and to keep them there.

CHAPTER 9

Games Kids and Parents Can Play Together

In this chapter, I list nearly two dozen games that parents and kids can play together in the time they have together, generally after dinner and on weekends or holidays. Some of these activities are played indoors; some outdoors; and some both indoors and outdoors, depending on weather conditions, availability of daylight, and other such factors. Nearly all the games promote the same general benefits: alertness; hand-to-eye coordination; cooperation; movement (either lateral, forward/backward, or both); and, most importantly, confidence and satisfaction. All these and other benefits relate in some way to the primary aim of my program, which is to get kids to become aware of the importance of getting their weight down if they're overweight, and of developing the discipline and desire to *keep* it down. In other words, instilling healthier eating and exercise patterns in them that will hopefully become standards they will continue to follow throughout their adolescent and adult lives.

GAMES TO GET YOUR KIDS (AND YOU) MOVING

Here then are some of my top suggestions for games that are best played with two or more people.

500

This game needs three or more kids and a ball (either a football or a base-ball are common). One person is the thrower, and everyone else clusters about throwing-distance away from the thrower. The thrower tosses the ball in the air toward everyone else and announces a number between 50 and 500, like this: "I've got 200 up for grabs." If a kid catches it they get as many points as the thrower yelled. If they drop it, though, they lose the same number of points (negative scores are possible).

The first person to get 500 points wins and become the thrower for the next game. Or, try this next variation.

One person is the thrower, and everyone else clusters about throwing-distance away from the thrower. The ball is then thrown (or kicked) toward the group. If caught on the fly, it is worth 100 points; after the first bounce, 75 points; after the second bounce, 50; and after the third bounce, 25.

The first person to reach 500 becomes the thrower (or kicker) for the next round.

Badminton

This is an old-favorite backyard game that the entire family can enjoy. Badminton sets can be purchased inexpensively at most sporting goods stores or in department store sports sections. A set consists of a net on poles that you drive into the ground; usually two to four racquets; and several shuttlecocks (commonly called birdies) that you hit back and forth over the net. A birdie has a rounded rubber tip with either feathers or thin plastic mesh arranged in a cone-shaped pattern, narrowing down at the tip. When you hit the birdie over the net with the racquet it always sails over to your partner with the weighted tip facing downward.

When you set up the net, make sure that the top of it is higher than the top of your head but not too high for your child. (However, if this proves to be a problem with your child, you may consider lowering it to just above their height to get them used to putting the birdie over the net, then gradually raise it as they improve.) The racquets are used to serve the birdie and to hit it back over the net; the same way they are in tennis.

Badminton can be played competitively, with rules and scorekeeping. I would suggest not doing this with your child—at least not in the beginning, anyway. The main thing you want to do is to get them used to just hitting the birdie and putting it over the net, developing their speed, hand-to-eye coordination, and confidence. Competitive play can come later but only if your child feels confident enough to do it. If you only have one child, one of you should be on his or her side of the net, helping them. If you have two children, one of them should be on each side of the net and one of you should be with each of them. Three or more children, work it out accordingly. But, however you do it, make sure that your child has ample opportunities to hit the birdie and attempt to put it over the net. Remember, you're doing this for them more than for yourselves. Step back and let them take their shot at it. If they miss or fail to put it over, just say "Oh well," and continue to encourage them. Sooner or later, with practice, they'll get it right.

Balloon Training

This is a great training tool for children who are not physically active or strong or well-coordinated. It is especially beneficial for young people who may have disabilities but have the use of their arms and hands.

Since balloons are so light, there is no real exertion involved as the kids hit the balloons back and forth, or hit them to each other and try to catch them before they hit the floor. For variation, they can try bouncing the balloons on their knees before hitting them back to their partners. There are as many variations of games that can be played with balloons as the children's imaginations can devise.

Studies such as the one published in the *Strength and Conditioning Journal* of the National Strength and Conditioning Association (August 2008) concluded that "balloon training can offer a safe and enjoyable method of improving selected measures of health and fitness in school-age youth with and without disabilities, provided that age-appropriate guidelines are followed."

Dodge Ball

This requires a long wall or side of a house or garage, and a big rubber ball or kick ball, as well as three or more people. All but one person lines up and the one person who doesn't throws the ball at the wall or siding in an attempt to hit a part of someone's body (in some variations you can only hit them below the waist). If they do, then that person is "it" and he or she must now throw the ball. The object is not to throw the ball hard, but to throw it accurately, in order to catch someone trying to dodge the ball. Or, try the following variation.

You can gather up a few of your neighbors and, if your group is large enough (say, a dozen players or more), you can play dodge ball in a circle, using roughly the same rules. There are two groups of equal numbers, one group in the circle and the other forming the circle on the outside. The players on the outside circle throw the ball at the players inside the circle, trying to hit them. The ball is thrown by whoever retrieves it when it is thrown by another player. When someone gets hit they have to leave the circle. When all the players who were inside the circle get hit and are eliminated, the two groups trade places. Dodge ball is a great game for learning and using lateral movement and coordination, as you attempt to literally "dodge" the ball as it is being thrown at you.

Down Down Down

This game comes to us from the land "Down Under," referring to Australia.

You start off with a tennis ball and choose up sides. If there are three of you (two adults and a child), one adult goes on the side with the child. If there are four of you (two kids and two adults) one adult pairs off with one child. Three or more kids, figure it out accordingly.

The two sides move a reasonable distance apart. You throw the ball continuously back and forth as fast as you can until somebody drops it. When someone drops the ball you say, "Down on one knee." The person who dropped the ball must then continue the game in that position. If the same person drops it a second time then you say, "Down on two knees." Then if the same person drops the ball again you say, "Down on one elbow." If they drop it a fourth time you say, "Down on two elbows," and a fifth time "Down on your chin." After that, you're out. But before you're eliminated, you have to stay in the position you're in to catch the ball and throw the ball.

Frisbee

Tossing a Frisbee around in the yard or the street (if it's not too busy) is another fun thing families can do. Sometimes you can even include your family dog. Many people train their dogs to catch the Frisbee and return it to them. Frisbees are relatively inexpensive and can be thrown a number of different ways. Traditionally, it is thrown sideways and it sails directly to the person you're aiming at, but you can add twists to it and throw it like a curve ball, or even a boomerang that will come back to you if you throw it on just the right angle high into the air.

There are a number of games you can play with a Frisbee. One of them is called Razorblade. A Frisbee and three or more players are needed. One person starts with the Frisbee and throws it wildly. All players decide whether to get the Frisbee or not. Usually, only the closest person will try to get it and the others run away from that person. Once the person has it, he or she yells to the others that he or she has it and the others freeze in place. They cannot move their feet, but can move all other body parts.

The person with the Frisbee is allowed to take three steps in any direction and then throw it at someone. If it hits the target person, then that person loses the use of that limb (for example, if it hits an arm or leg), or dies if it hits their torso. The Frisbee acts like a "razorblade," "cutting off" the limb or "killing" the person. If the target person catches the Frisbee, then they can either get a limb back or take one from the thrower. The target person then may throw it at another person. If a thrower misses, then everyone may run until someone picks up the Frisbee. The last person "alive" wins.

Hopscotch

Parents and kids can both have fun
playing this. Following the classic
diagram at right, you can draw a
hopscotch board on your driveway
with washable, removable chalk.
Each square should be about 18 to
24 inches in both height and width.
(For indoor play, masking tape can
be used on a wood or cement floor.)

Each player has a marker (or
potsy) such as a stone, beanbag,
bottle cap, seashell, or button. The
first player stands behind the starting line to toss his or her marker in
square one. He or she hops on one
foot over square one to square two,
then continues hopping to square
eight, turns around, and hops back
again. He or she pauses in square
two to pick up the marker, hops
in square one, and then out. Then
he or she continues by tossing the
marker in square two. All hopping
is done on one foot unless the
hopscotch design is such that two
squares are side-by-side. Then two
feet can be placed down with one in

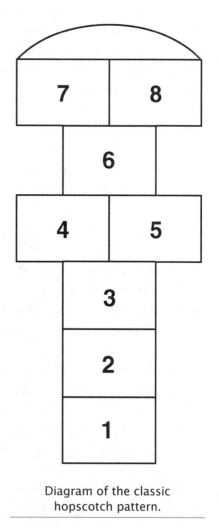

Diagram of the classic
hopscotch pattern.

each square. A player must always hop over any square where a marker
has been placed.

A player is out if: 1) the marker fails to land in the proper square;
2) the hopper steps on a line or out of bounds; 3) the hopper loses balance
when bending over to pick up the marker and puts a second hand or foot
down; 4) the hopper goes into a square where a marker is; or 5) they

put two feet down in a single box. The player puts the marker in the square where he or she will resume playing on the next turn, and the next player begins.

Sometimes a dome-shaped "rest area" is added on one end of the hopscotch pattern where the player can rest for a second or two and turn around before hopping back through.

Jump Rope

This is one of the simplest, least costly, combination game and exercise for both kids and their parents. All that's needed is a length of rope. It must be long enough to pass safely over your head and under your feet without having to stoop too much, if you're jumping rope as an individual. Or it can be longer, if a parent is holding each end and the kid is jumping in the middle. While you are jumping rope with your kids you can make it even more fun by reciting rhymes. There is a whole list of them to be found at the website www.gameskidsplay.net/jump_rope_ryhmes/index.htm.

King of the Hill (or Mountain)

This game can be played with several players and a mound or hill of dirt, or a large, low-cut tree stump. One person is chosen at random to be King of the Hill. Then, one at a time or in groups of two, each player goes up the hill to "dethrone" the King. The object is to get the king off of the hill by pushing or pulling or trickery. (No rough stuff, though; be careful that no one gets hurt.) There is no ultimate winner in this game—just a lot of fun. Especially when one of the kids dethrones mom or dad!

Running Bases

The rules of this game are pretty simple. You'll need two bases (old rugs, cardboard squares, base-sized linoleum squares, ceiling tiles, or anything similar will do); a softball; and two softball gloves. Or, if you don't have gloves, just use a ball that's not "hard" like a tennis ball or an ordinary rubber ball. Three people are required: two throwers—preferably mom and dad—and a runner, their child.

Set up the two bases about twenty feet apart. Each parent stands in front of each of the bases and one kid at a time takes his or her turn on the bases. The parents toss the ball back and forth and, at some point, the child must run toward the opposite base. They must not stay on the base for more than three tosses or they lose points. (*Hint to kids:* begin running when the parent at the opposite base throws the ball to the parent on the base nearest you.) The object is for the child to make it safely to the opposite base without getting tagged out by the parent with the ball (sliding may be allowable if played on a soft surface like a lawn).

The child gets a point for each base they reach safely before being tagged out. If the ball is thrown wide by one parent and gets past the other, the child can run back and forth and take as many bases as they can get away with. If the child is caught in a rundown between their parents, they can attempt to run around them as long as they don't run out of bounds on either side of the base path, which should be clearly marked. If the parent drops the ball while tagging the child, the child automatically takes the next base and gets a point for it. Parents who have their kids in a rundown cannot advance past the midway point between the bases while attempting to tag the child. If they do, the child gets to take the next base. When the child is tagged out they keep track of their points and the next child takes a base and begins to play, continuing until they are tagged out. The game is over after the last child has their turn. The child with the highest number of points is the winner.

Other Tag Games

Many, if not most of us, parents played some sort of "Tag! You're it!" games when we were kids. There are so many variations of tag, there isn't enough space here to list them all. The big advantage of tag is that it can be played outdoors or indoors.

The most traditional and common form of tag has one person ("it"), chosen in some prearranged manner (drawing straws, shooting "odd or even" fingers toward each other, etc.), closing their eyes and counting to a certain number—usually fifty. The other players will hide somewhere and the person who is "it" will begin searching for them when they finish counting and opens their eyes.

Those who are in hiding must leave their hiding places (when they think they won't be seen), and run toward a pre-designated "base" and reach it safely without being tagged by the person who is "it." Anyone who is tagged before reaching the base, or is found still in their hiding place, then becomes "it." If everyone gets safely to base, the same person is "it" again.

The person who is "it" cannot be a "base sticker." They must actively search for those in hiding and not just wait by the base for everyone to run to it. Likewise, none of the other players can be a "base sticker" either. They cannot wait next to the base while the one who is "it" is counting, then touch the base safely when the "it" person opens their eyes. When a person touches the base before they are tagged, they call out, "Safe!" If they are tagged before reaching the base, the one tagging them calls out, "Tag! You're It!" The game ends when the first person is tagged, then that person becomes "it" and a new round begins.

For or a list of other tag games, go to www.gameskidsplay.net/games/chasing_games/index.htm.

SPORTS PREPARATION GAMES (FUNDAMENTALS)

For parents hoping to get their child interested in playing competitive sports, as well as for the child who may want to go into any of these sports, there are ways they can prep for all of them in or around their own homes. Competitive sports are good for children in ways that are almost incalculable. It helps them develop physically and mentally, and the levels of activity involved are conducive to helping control their weight. Below is a listing of my suggestions for prepping your child for some of our most popular sports.

Baseball Pitch and Catch (or Batting)

This is good preparation for getting the kids into playing baseball. All you need are balls, gloves, and bats. You can start by placing yourself a reasonable distance from your child and throwing a ball back and forth and catching it. (Be sure to stay within a distance your child can throw.) This gives them the basics on throwing the ball and catching it. You can throw them "line drives" or "pop-ups," then possibly switch them over to actually "pitching" the ball over a "plate" that you squat behind and play catcher. Start with a softball, then gradually move them up to a hardball when they are ready.

If you have a big enough yard or driveway, you can then get them into some batting fundamentals, using a softball or Wiffle ball that won't break any windows if hit too hard. Dad or mom can pitch and the other can catch and, while one kid is batting, the other(s) can play the field or the bases, if you want to give them running practice after they hit the ball. The kids take turns batting and fielding. You can instruct your child on how to bunt or swing away and how to slide into bases. Once they have the fundamentals down pat and if they have the desire, you can sign them up for a team on your local playground or Little League or at school.

Basketball

This is also a sport either boys or girls can play in your driveway at home. Full basketball goals with the stand, net, and backboard can be costly and, unless you're budgeted for it, you don't have to feel obligated to provide it. For less money, you can buy just the net and backboard and mount it on your garage or carport. However, if that's too high for your child, you can mount it on the side of the garage or carport at a height more suitable for them, later moving the basket up higher as they get better and taller. If you don't want to spend any money on baskets, though, you can use a large, open container like a metal storage drum, an open plastic storage container stacked on other storage containers, or even a stack of old car tires. Whichever method you choose, the objective is to teach your child how to shoot toward a target with an opening into which they can sink the ball. Like all the other sports, once they get proficient at shooting baskets, they may want you to sign them up for team play.

Football Tossing/Kicking

As in pitch and catch, this is a good way to get your son(s) into football. You simply pass the ball back and forth, giving him practice in both throwing and catching. You might even add running to the game, allowing him to run toward you and a "goal line" after he catches the ball. If you have the yard space, you might even do a little kicking and receiving. But you may want to start with a soft football at first, then work your way up to a harder one.

If your child shows an interest in the game, you may want to determine which position he would like to play after explaining to him what each position entails. If he wants to play a line position, either offense or defense, practice the position with him. If he wants to be a running back, give him the ball and let him run with it. If he wants to be a pass receiver, have him stand next to you while you have the ball, count to three or five, have him run forward, then throw the ball to him. Later, when you and he feel ready, you can sign him up for a playground or league or school team.

Golf

You can teach your child, boy or girl, the fundamentals of golf using either a play set of plastic clubs and balls or a set of basic clubs that are an appropriate length for their height. But only use plastic balls unless you are on a driving range or an actual course, which should only come later, when your kids are ready. Real golf balls are very hard and can do personal harm or property damage, especially in close quarters. You can set up a net in your backyard and have your child hit the plastic practice balls against it, using a variety of woods and irons, with the balls teed up and on the ground. You can also give them practice putting by setting a target and designating it as the "hole." Indoors you can help your kid practice putting on the carpet, allowing them to hit the ball softly toward a cup or a box turned on its side into which they "sink" it.

Gymnastics

Gymnastics covers a wide range of physical activities that challenge the body and its component parts in many ways. The simplest things you and your child can do are tumbling activities, either on an interior carpet or on the lawn, preferably on blankets. You may want to add some extra padding just to be on the safe side, and foam rubber-filled plastic mats are inexpensive. You and your child can do handstands, again on the padded carpet or lawn, or even cartwheels if you have the room. Some backyard swing sets have "chinning bars" for doing pull-ups or seesaws, which are good for developing leg muscles. If you use your imagination you can come up with different things you and your child can do to limber up your bodies with gymnastics. And, of course, if your child shows a proclivity toward any particular gymnastic specialty or specialties, you can enroll them in a gymnastics program at school, the local playground, or a commercial facility. Just be careful about certain gymnastic activities at home and, parents, be sure to "spot" for your kids to prevent them from injuring themselves.

Soccer

Boys or girls can do this game with their parents. Take an ordinary soccer ball and place it on the ground, kicking it back and forth between you. Then try some actual running moves, moving the ball along with your toes or the sides of your feet. As you move the ball toward your child or vice versa, each of you can try to block the other or steal the ball. You can set up goals on either side of the yard that are simply lines you have to kick the ball over. Later on, you can show your child how to move or stop the ball with other parts of the body that are legal in regulation soccer, making sure they don't use their hands. You can even set your child up as a goalie and have them practice stopping the ball that you either throw or kick toward them, while allowing them the use of their hands. Later, if they feel ready, you can enroll them in a playground or league program, or in their school's team if they have one.

Tennis

Few of us are wealthy enough to have our own tennis courts but that shouldn't stop those who have an interest in learning the game. Sometimes all it takes is a hard wall and a paved surface in front of it. You and your child can practice hitting a tennis ball or other soft ball against the wall with your racquets. It's like having another player hitting the ball back to you. You can teach your child forehand strokes, backhand, and other strokes used during a competitive tennis match. Later, if they show an interest in the game, you can set up a regular once- or twice-a-week routine to go to a local tennis court. (They are usually free on neighborhood playgrounds or, at most, a nominal fee may be charged.) There you can practice serving and hitting the ball over the net. Don't keep score unless your child feels proficient enough to play competitively against you. The main object is to get them hitting the ball consistently over the net and learning coordination. For developing movement—both lateral and forward/backward, as well as hand-to-eye coordination—there are few sports or games better than tennis.

OLD-TIME FAVORITES

Here are a few other games that were popular when I was a kid that parents and their kids today can play if they can gather up a few other parents and kids from the neighborhood. They are also popular at large gatherings such as birthday parties and family reunions.

Crack the Whip

You need at least six people for the game to be effective, but the more the better. You also need a fairly large area like a big yard or a park. You all hold hands as you would for Red Rover (see next), but there is only one line. Someone is picked to be the leader (head of the whip) and someone else as the tail, preferably a parent in each case. The leader just starts running around in whip-like patterns, zigzagging, and swerving side to side.

Everyone else follows, being sure not to let go of hands. Usually, after everyone has been running at full speed and making sharp turns, the tail and/or people next to him or her get sent flying because of the force of everyone running and turning. This is a lot of fun but be prepared to get dirty if you're on the end. The head and the tail of the whip can use two hands to hold on to the one person they are connected to. The tail tries as hard as they can to not let go. (Holding on and being whipped around is usually funnier then letting go and rolling to a stop.)

Red Rover

In this game, there are two opposing lines and members of one line attempt to "break through" the opposing team's line. At first, two teams are chosen of equal size (at least five on each side, but the more the better), and they form two lines, facing each other and holding hands. One side starts by picking a person on the opposing team and saying "Red Rover, Red Rover, send _____ (person's name) right over."

The person named lets go of his teammates and begins a headlong rush for the other line. Their goal is to break through the line by overpowering their opponents' hold on each other or by sneaking under their linked hands. If that person breaks through, they choose one person from the opposing team to join their team, and they both go back and join in their line. If they fail to break through, that person becomes part of the other team. Each team alternates calling people over until one team has all the people and is declared the winner.

Steal the Bacon

In this game you have two opposing lines facing each other, about twenty to thirty feet apart. Midway between the lines is an object designated as the "bacon." The object of Steal the Bacon is to take the bacon back to your own side without being caught. The bacon can be almost anything: a glove, a ball or, best yet if someone has one—a bowling pin. One person, an adult, must be designated as the umpire or scorekeeper.

The members of each team are numbered. The umpire then calls out a number, preferably at random. The players on each side who are assigned that number run toward the bacon. No other team members leave their side of the field. If the player on one side is faster and arrives at the bacon sooner than the other, he or she must wait by the bacon until the other player arrives. At that point, the two players begin their attempt to steal the bacon without getting caught (tagged).

The two opposing players will often hover over the bacon or circle around it, faking grabs at it with either hand—feinting, then pulling away without touching the object—waiting for a slight advantage to grab it and run back before the other player can react. Neither player may tag or touch the other until one of them actually "steals" the bacon and starts to run off with it. If the player stealing the bacon successfully carries it back over to his or her own side, their team scores a point. (*Variation:* in some games, points are scored by carrying it to the other team's side or either team's side.)

If a player is tagged after stealing the bacon before he or she returns to their own side, the team that tagged him or her scores a point. The umpire is keeping score, which can be announced after each "round." The game is over when a predetermined number of points are scored, or when all numbers have been called.

WHAT PARENTS CAN DO

In the interests of their child's health and fitness, parents should commit themselves to family time spent playing together, and they should be receptive to the games or sports in which their child shows interest and/or proficiency. It may be all too easy for parents to attempt to cop out if they are tired at the end of a long workday, but the effort should be made anyway—for the benefit of the child if not for themselves. During the course of such play, it is very likely that their kid's talents might come to the forefront and the parents can then begin steering them in that direction. If they show a love and proclivity toward football or soccer or tennis or some other competitive sport, the parents can work with them on their skills or enroll them in the youth sports program of their choice. And, above all, parents shouldn't discourage their children from pursuing a sport or activity they seem to enjoy but aren't particularly good at. They shouldn't berate them if they are clumsy or uncoordinated. Patience and persistence are the keys to your child's happiness and success—as well as your own.

There are many other games that can be beneficial to both parents and their children and they can be found on a number of reputable, reliable websites. You can find these websites using popular search engines like Google or America Online (if you're an AOL subscriber) and typing in the key words "children's games." One of the most comprehensive sources is Kids Games at www.gameskidsplay.net, which supplied much of the material in this chapter. But there are other good sites, which are listed in the Resources section.

As an added word of advice, always check with your child's physician to determine his or her ability to take part in physical activities. He or she will know what's best for your child.

Good luck and—above all—have fun!

CHAPTER 9 SUMMARY

- Simple games that can be played inside or outside can be used as a source of exercise for the whole family.

- Teaching your family how to incorporate fun activities into their lifestyle will aid in the desire to be physically active on a daily basis.

- Allowing a child to be part of the development of the game format and rules will ultimately vest the child in the outcome, while not singling out the child, as the target game.

- Games also allow for the emotional and physical development of the child with emphasis on creative imagery, gross motor skill development, and problem solving in a group setting—all critical components of the proper childhood and maturation process.

PART FIVE

Tracking Tools and
Resource Guide
for a Fitter,
Leaner Child

CHAPTER 10

Body Plan for Kids
A Day-by-Day Nutritional and Activity Guide

Now that we have discussed the overall problems of childhood obesity, its most common causes, and what can be done to combat the condition, it is time to start putting what you have learned so far into practice with your kids and yourselves, since you, as their parents, are the key to making the Body Plan for Kids work for them. You are your kids' coaches, mentors, and examples you want to encourage them to follow.

In this chapter and on my website (www.BodyPlanForKids.com), you will find helpful tools for preparing your child or children for the job that lies ahead of them in losing pounds and keeping them off. Or, if they're not overweight, how to keep them from reaching that point. These tracking tools include illustrations such as weekly fitness and nutritional scorecards, charts, and other helpful guidelines that can get you and your kids on the right path to weight loss and overall fitness.

Let me just summarize with some of the basics, as outlined below.

STEP 1

If you have not done so already, get accurate height and weight measurements using the instructions previously provided in Chapter 3.

STEP 2

If you have not done so already, determine your child's body mass index and fat-to-lean-muscle ratio, using the instructions provided in Chapter 3. Remember to check your child's BMI and fat-to-lean-muscle ratio once a week.

STEP 3

If you have not done so already, make an appointment to consult with your family doctor to confirm your verdict that your child, yourself, or any other family member may be overweight. Work with your doctor to determine the proper goal weight for all concerned and before beginning a new fitness or nutrition regimen.

STEP 4

Once you've visited your health-care provider to get started on the right plan for yourself and your child, I can help you by providing the resources to start solving the problem. No plan is complete without a way to track your progress. Once you've registered your family team, it's time to start tracking! The "Weight Tracker" tool lets you:

- Register as many family members as you like.
- Track your family's eating and exercise habits.
- Track weekly weight loss.
- Upload photos to keep track of "visible" progress.
- See quick stats.
- Graph of weight-loss progress.

To pull up these tools or to print them out, log on to www.bodyplan forkids.com/wt. (You must be registered with the site and have a username and password to log in with. If you're not, you can register and create a password the first time you log in. There is no charge to register.) Once you enter the site you will find nine horizontal blue boxes labeled in the following categories: Home, This Week's Weight, Food Diary, Weight-Loss Graph, Printable Chart, Photo Updates, Exercise Diary, Stats Page, and Administration. Click on the box you are interested in printing out or using to record your data on. Or, instead of printing them out, you can enter the information directly onto the website and track your child's progress there electronically. Some of the most important tools you will need are shown on the following pages.

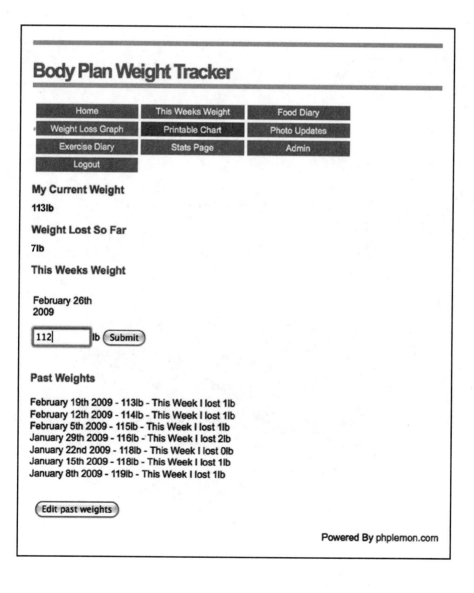

Body Plan Weight Tracker

Home	This Weeks Weight	Food Diary
Weight Loss Graph	Printable Chart	Photo Updates
Exercise Diary	Stats Page	Admin
Logout		

My Current Weight

112lb

Weight Lost So Far

8lb

Exercise Diary

Friday February 26th 2009

Played kickball in PE today (1 hour)

Walked around block a few times with mom after school (45 minutes)

10 pushups and stretched (15 minutes)

Edit This Page

You can update this days exercise diary by clicking the button below.

(Add/Edit/Delete)

Powered By phplemon.com

Weight Loss Graph

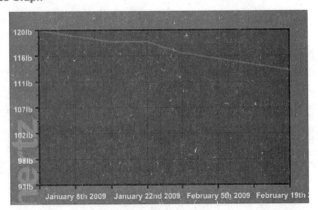

Powered By phplemon.com

Body Plan Weight Tracker

Home	This Weeks Weight	Food Diary
Weight Loss Graph	Printable Chart	Photo Updates
Exercise Diary	Stats Page	Admin
Logout		

My Current Weight

112lb

Weight Lost So Far

8lb

Printable Chart

Printable Version - Click Here

120lb	119lb	118lb	117lb	116lb	115lb	114lb	113lb	112lb						

Powered By phplemon.com

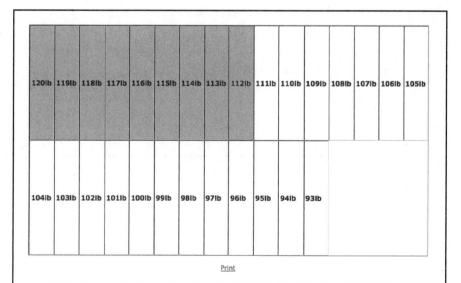

120lb	119lb	118lb	117lb	116lb	115lb	114lb	113lb	112lb	111lb	110lb	109lb	108lb	107lb	106lb	105lb
104lb	103lb	102lb	101lb	100lb	99lb	98lb	97lb	96lb	95lb	94lb	93lb				

Print

Body Plan Weight Tracker

Home	This Weeks Weight	Food Diary
Weight Loss Graph	Printable Chart	Photo Updates
Exercise Diary	Stats Page	Admin
Logout		

My Current Weight

112lb

Weight Lost So Far

8lb

Food Diary

Friday February 26th 2009

2 scrambled eggs, 1 slice of whole wheat toast, 1 Tsp sugar free jelly, 6 grapes, and 1 cup of skim milk

10 whole grain crackers, few slices of turkey meat, 1 slice of cheese, 1 orange, water

Grilled chicken, spinach, wheat pasta (the size of a baseball), 1 cup of skim milk

After school snack: banana and peanut butter with water

Edit This Page

You can Add more foods, edit foods or delete foods from this day in your **Food Diary**, by clicking the button below.

(Add/Edit/Delete)

Powered By phplemon.com

Body Plan Weight Tracker

Home	This Weeks Weight	Food Diary
Weight Loss Graph	Printable Chart	Photo Updates
Exercise Diary	Stats Page	Admin
Logout		

My Current Weight
112lb

Weight Lost So Far
8lb

Stats

Target Weight (as determined in conjunction with your healthcare practitioner)
93lb

Weight Lost So Far
8lb

Weight Lost In Last Week
1lb

Weight Lost In Last Month
3lb

Highest Weekly Weight Loss
2lb - January 29th 2009

myWEIGHT
112lb
50.85kg

Powered By phplemon.com

Body Plan Weight Tracker

Home	This Weeks Weight	Food Diary
Weight Loss Graph	Printable Chart	Photo Updates
Exercise Diary	Stats Page	Admin
Logout		

My Current Weight

112lb

Weight Lost So Far

8lb

Admin

You must press 'Submit' after every option that you have selected.

Start Weight

| 120 | lb (Submit)

Target Weight

| 93 | lb (Submit)

First Weigh In Date

[1st ▲▼] [January ▲▼] [2009 ▲▼] (Submit)

Weekly Weight Update Day

Monday   ○
Tuesday   ○
Wednesday   ○
Thursday   ○
Friday   ●
Saturday   ○
Sunday   ○

(Submit)

Weight Input Type

● Use default input type
○ Pounds Only (lbs)

(Submit)

Reset Database

(Submit)

Powered By phplemon.com

WHAT PARENTS CAN DO

For parents who have read this book, the information on my website can be used as the next step in the weight loss/maintenance process. It can serve as a support network for discipline and motivation, along with other individuals with whom the child may have a strong relationship, such as grandparents, aunts, uncles, other family members, and friends. The child who is trying to lose weight and become more fit needs to know that he or she isn't in this quest alone.

In addition to these charts and diaries, my Body Plan for Kids website is a resource for other vital information about nutrition, weight loss, and exercise and activity for youngsters and their families. Through some of these links, you can access articles on these subjects, studies that have been performed, and the latest news and research on childhood obesity. I have assembled a team of experts, some of whom assisted me in the writing of this book with their firsthand knowledge, and they will be able to answer many of the questions you might have. I've even had my nutritionist, Julie Fortenberry, post some menus, recipes, and lists of healthy foods and snacks, including some from my previous books.

We are now offering video clips from East Jefferson General Hospital's "Healthy Lifestyles" segments with tips and educational information on exercise, nutrition, and healthy lifestyle choices. You can even join our Parents Forum at www.BodyPlanForKids.com, which will allow you to post helpful comments you may want to share about how the Body Plan for Kids is working for you and your children. And, if you and/or your business wish to become one of my Body Plan Partners, please contact me. I would welcome your support and participation.

Yet another added benefit I am offering to Body Plan participants—and others—is free access to my health tips, for which you can register on the site by logging on to my home page at www.BodyPlanForKids.com/index.php or www.mackieshilstone.com. In these tips, I present up-to-date information for the whole family. It's called "MackieMail." I also invite your comments on all childhood obesity-related subjects, and offer a forum for posting any comments and questions you may have. I am pleased to answer all questions that are directed toward me, and I will answer them to the best of my knowledge, consulting with my experts when necessary.

You can email me through the site at www.BodyPlanForKids.com/profiles.php?uid=6, or even e-mail me directly at mackie@mackieshilstone.com.

If you'd like to reach me by phone or mail, my contact information is:

> Mackie Shilstone's Body Plan for Kids
> 2901 Magazine Street
> New Orleans, LA 70130
> Phone: (504) 897-1030
> Fax: (504) 897-1050

In closing, I want to wish all of you parents and children the best of luck as you pursue your weight loss and fitness goals. As I've said, becoming fit and staying fit is the job of a lifetime. Healthy, active kids tend to become healthy, active adults, and we need healthy adults to guide our nation in the generations to come. I hope my Body Plan for Kids program has been helpful for you and I certainly welcome your feedback.

CHAPTER 10 SUMMARY

- Keeping track of your child's weight, height, food/beverage intake, and exercise is essential in helping to maintain a healthy weight and lifestyle.

- Maintain a daily food and activity log, such as appears in this chapter or on the www.BodyPlanForKids.com website, for the whole family to help identify areas for improvement.

APPENDIX A

Expert Committee Recommendations

On the Assessment, Prevention, and Treatment of Child and Adolescent Overweight and Obesity

Throughout this book I often refer to the American Medical Association (AMA) Expert Committee on the Assessment, Prevention, and Treatment of Child and Adolescent Overweight and Obesity, a landmark report drafted in January 2007 that identified new treatment and prevention options to address the growing problem of overweight and obese children. This report is published in full below. The recommendations target the eight- to twelve-year-old group (the focus of this book), as well as those in the thirteen- to eighteen-year-old group.

Assessment Recommendations

1. The Expert Committee recommends that physicians and allied health-care providers perform, at a minimum, a yearly assessment of weight status in all children, and that this assessment include calculation of height, weight (measured appropriately), and body mass index (BMI) for age and plotting of those measures on standard growth charts.

2. With regard to classification, the Expert Committee recommends that:

   a. Individuals from the ages of two to eighteen years, with a BMI > 95th percentile for age and sex, or a BMI exceeding 30 (whichever is smaller), should be considered obese.

   b. Individuals with a BMI > 85th percentile, but < 95th percentile for age and sex, should be considered overweight, and this term replaces "at risk of overweight."

3. The Expert Committee recommends use of the 99th percentile of BMI for age cut-offs (indicate by using a table with cut-points for the 99th percentile BMI by age and gender) to allow for improved accessibility of the data in the clinical setting and for additional study.

4. The Expert Committee recommends against routine clinical use of skinfold thickness in the assessment of obesity in children.

5. The Expert Committee was unable to recommend the use of waist circumference for routine clinical use at the present time because of incomplete information and lack of specific guidance for clinical application.

6. The Expert Committee recommends that qualitative assessment of dietary patterns of all pediatric patients be conducted, at a minimum, at each well child visit for anticipatory guidance, and that assessment include the following areas:

   a. Self-efficacy and readiness to change.

   b. Identification of the following specific dietary practices, which may be targets for change:

      i. Frequency of eating outside the home at restaurants or fast food establishments.

      ii. Excessive consumption of sweetened beverages.

      iii. Consumption of excessive portion sizes for age.

   c. Additional practices to be considered for evaluation during the qualitative dietary assessment include:

      i. Excessive consumption of 100 percent fruit juice.

      ii. Breakfast consumption (frequency and quality).

      iii. Excessive consumption of foods that are high in energy density.

      iv. Low consumption of fruits and vegetables.

      v. Meal frequency and snacking patterns (including quality).

7. The Expert Committee recommends that assessment of levels of physical activity and sedentary behaviors should be performed in all pediatric patients at a minimum, at each well child visit for anticipatory guidance, and should include these general areas:

   a. Self-efficacy and readiness to change.

   b. Environment and social support and barriers to physical activity.

   c. Whether the child is meeting recommendations of sixty minutes of at least moderate physical activity per day.

   d. Level of sedentary behavior, which should include hours of behavior such as television and/or DVD watching, playing video games, and using the computer, and comparison to a baseline of < 2 hours per day.

8. The Expert Committee recommends that physicians and other allied health-care providers obtain a focused family history for obesity, type 2 diabetes, cardiovascular disease (particularly hypertension), and early deaths from heart disease or stroke to assess risk of current or future comorbidities associated with a child's overweight or obese status.

9. The Expert Committee recommends a thorough physical examination and that for a child identified as overweight or obese, the following areas be included in addition to the aforementioned recommendations on BMI:

   a. Waist circumference is increasingly being invoked as an indicator of insulin resistance and other comorbidities of obesity, and may be useful to characterize risk in the obese child. Because of the difficulty in measuring and the uncertainty of appropriate cut-offs, however, routine use is not recommended at this time.

   b. Pulse.

      i. Measured in the standard pediatric manner.

   c. Blood pressure.

      i. Measured with a large enough cuff so that 80 percent of the arm is covered by the bladder of the cuff.

d. Signs associated with comorbidities of overweight and obesity.

10. The Expert Committee recommends that the following laboratory tests be considered in the evaluation of a child identified as overweight or obese:

a. If the BMI for age and sex is:

i. 85th to 94th percentile with no risk factors: fasting lipid profile.

ii. 85th to 94th percentile with risk factors in history or physical examination, obtain in addition: aspartate aminotransferase (AST) and alanine aminotransferase (ALT), fasting glucose.

iii. Greater than the 95th percentile, even in the absence of risk factors: all the tests listed under ii, plus blood urea nitrogen (BUN), and creatinine.

b. Guidelines for laboratory assessment and testing are also provided for more detailed evaluation, typically performed and interpreted by subspecialists.

Treatment Recommendations

1. The Expert Committee recommends that all physicians and healthcare providers should address weight management and lifestyle issues with all patients regardless of presenting weight, at a minimum, each year.

2. The Expert Committee recommends that all children between two and eighteen years of age with a BMI between the 5th and 84th percentile should follow the recommendations for prevention as outlined in the Prevention Recommendations.

3. The Expert Committee recommends that the treatment of overweight children be approached in a staged method based upon the child's age, BMI, any related comorbidities, weight status of parents, and progress in treatment, and that the child's primary caregivers/families be involved in the process.

4. The Expert Committee recommends the following staged approach for children between the ages of two and nineteen years and whose BMI is above the 85th percentile:

   a. Stage 1. Prevention Plus Protocol: These recommendations can be implemented by the primary care physician or allied health-care provider who has some training in pediatric weight management/behavioral counseling. Stage 1 recommendations include:

      i. Dietary habits and physical activity:

        1. Five or more servings of fruits and vegetables per day.

        2. Two or fewer hours of screen time per day, and no television in the room where the child sleeps.

        3. One hour or more of daily physical activity.

        4. No sugar-sweetened beverages.

      ii. Patients and families of the patient be counseled to facilitate these eating behaviors:

        1. Eating a daily breakfast.

        2. Limiting meals outside of the home.

        3. Family meals should happen at least five to six times per week.

        4. Allowing the child to self-regulate his or her meals and avoiding overly restrictive behaviors.

      iii. Within this category, the goal should be weight maintenance with growth that results in a decreasing BMI as age increases.

        1. Monthly follow-up.

      iv. After three to six months, if no improvement in BMI/weight status has been noted, advancement to Stage 2 is indicated and based on patient/family readiness to change.

   b. Stage 2. Structured Weight Management Protocol. These recommendations can be implemented by a primary care physician or allied health-care provider highly trained in weight management. Stage 2 recommendations include:

      i. Dietary and physical activity behaviors.

1. Development of a plan for utilization of a balanced macronutrient diet emphasizing low amounts of energy-dense foods.
2. Increased structured daily meals and snacks.
3. Supervised active play of at least sixty minutes per day.
4. Screen time of one hour or less per day.
5. Increased monitoring (e.g., screen time, physical activity, dietary intake, restaurant logs) by provider, patient and/or family.

ii. Within this category, goal should be weight maintenance that results in a decreasing BMI as age and height increases; however, weight loss should not exceed 1 lb/month in children aged two to eleven years, or an average of 2 lb/week in older overweight/obese children and adolescents.

iii. If no improvement in BMI/weight after three to six months, patient should be advanced to Stage 3.

c. Stage 3. Comprehensive Multidisciplinary Protocol. At this level of intervention, the patient should optimally be referred to a multidisciplinary obesity care team.

i. Eating and activity goals are the same as in Stage 2.

ii. Activities within this category should also include:
1. Structured behavioral modification program, including food and activity monitoring and development of short-term diet and physical activity goals.
2. Involvement of primary caregivers/families for behavioral modification in children under age twelve years and training of primary caregivers/families for all children.

iii. Within this category, goal should be weight maintenance or gradual weight loss until BMI less than 85th percentile and should not exceed 1 lb/month in children aged two to five years, or 2 lbs/week in older obese children and adolescents.

5. The Expert Committee recommends the following for children with a BMI > 95th percentile, with significant comorbidities and who have not been successful with Stages 1 to 3, or children [with a BMI] > 99th

percentile, who have shown no improvement under Stage 3 (Comprehensive Multidisciplinary Intervention):

d. Stage 4. Tertiary Care Protocol. Referral to pediatric tertiary-weight management center with access to a multidisciplinary team with expertise in childhood obesity and which operates under a designed protocol.

   i. This protocol should include continued diet and activity counseling and the consideration of such additions as meal replacement, very-low-calorie diet, medication, and surgery.

6. The Expert Committee recommends that the following weight-loss targets should be considered when implementing the staged treatment plan:

a. Age Two to Five Years

   i. 85th–94th BMI: Weight maintenance until BMI < 85th percentile or slowing of weight gain as indicated by downward deflection in BMI curve.

   ii. > 95th BMI: Weight maintenance until BMI < 85th percentile; however, if weight loss occurs with a healthy and adequate caloric diet it should not exceed 1 lb/month. If greater loss is noted, monitor for causes of excessive weight loss.

   iii. BMI (> 21 or 22): (Rare, very high). Gradual weight loss not to exceed 1 lb/month. If greater loss occurs, monitor for causes of excessive weight loss.

b. Age Six to Eleven Years

   i. 85th–94th BMI: Weight maintenance until BMI < 85th percentile or slowing of weight gain as indicated by downward deflection in BMI curve.

   ii. 95th–98th BMI: Weight maintenance until BMI < 85th or gradual weight loss of approximately 1 lb/month. If greater loss is noted, monitor for causes of excessive weight loss.

   iii. > 99th BMI: Weight loss not to exceed an average of 2 lbs/week. If greater loss is noted, monitor for causes of excessive weight loss.

    c. Age Twelve to Eighteen Years

        i. 85th–94th BMI: Weight maintenance until BMI < 85th percentile, or slowing of weight gain as indicated by downward deflection in BMI curve.

       ii. 95th–98th BMI: Weight loss until BMI < 85th percentile—no more than an average of 2 lbs/week. If greater loss is noted, monitor for causes of excessive weight loss.

      iii. > 99th BMI: Weight loss not to exceed an average of 2 lbs/week. If greater loss is noted, monitor for causes of excessive weight loss.

7. The Expert Committee recommends that in children aged twelve to eighteen years, with BMI greater than the 99th percentile, primary care physicians and other allied health-care providers may begin treatment with Stages 1, 2, or 3 as indicated based on patient/family readiness to change.

Prevention Recommendations

1. The Expert Committee recommends that physicians and allied health-care providers counsel the following:

    a. For children aged two to eighteen years whose BMI is at or above the 5th percentile and no greater than the 84th percentile:

        i. Dietary intake:

          1. Limiting consumption of sugar-sweetened beverages and encouraging consumption of diets with recommended quantities of fruits and vegetables.

       ii. Physical activity:

          1. Limiting television and other screen time to one or two hours per day in children starting as young as age five years, as advised by the American Academy of Pediatrics and removing television and computer screens from children's primary sleeping area.

    iii. Eating behaviors:
       1. Eat breakfast daily.
       2. Limit eating out at restaurants, particularly fast food restaurants.
       3. Encourage family meals in which parents and children eat together.
       4. Limit portion size.

2. The Expert Committee recommends that physicians, allied health-care professionals, and professional organizations advocate for:

   a. The federal government to increase physical activity at school through intervention programs as early as grade 1 through the end of high school and college, and through creating school environments that support physical activity in general.

   b. Supporting efforts to preserve and enhance parks as areas for physical activity, informing local development initiatives regarding the inclusion of walking and bicycle paths, and promoting families' use of local physical activity options by making information and suggestions about physical activity alternatives available in doctors' offices.

3. The Expert Committee recommends using the following techniques to aid physicians and allied health-care providers who may wish to support obesity prevention in clinical, school, and community settings:

   a. Actively engage families with parental obesity or maternal diabetes, because these children are at increased risk for developing obesity even if they currently have a normal BMI.

   b. Encourage an authoritative* parenting style in support of increased physical activity and reduced sedentary behavior, providing tangible and motivational support for children.

---

* Authoritative parents are both demanding and responsive. "They monitor and impart clear standards for their children's conduct. They are assertive, but not intrusive and restrictive. Their disciplinary methods are supportive, rather than punitive. They want their children to be assertive as well as socially responsible, and self-regulated as well as cooperative" (Baumrind, 1991, p. 62).

   c. Discourage a restrictive** parenting style regarding child eating.

   d. Encourage parents to model healthy diets and portion sizes, physical activity, and limited television time.

   e. Promote physical activity at school and in child-care settings (including after school programs), by asking children and parents about activity in these settings during routine office visits.

4. The Expert Committee suggests that children of healthy weight participate in sixty minutes of moderate to vigorous physical activity daily.

   a. The sixty minutes can be accumulated throughout the day, as opposed to only single or long bouts.

   b. Ideally, such activity should be enjoyable to the child.

   c. Whereas some health and psychological benefits may be attained by achieving the sixty-minute goal, greater duration should yield increased benefit.

5. The Expert Committee also suggests counseling patients and families to perform these behaviors:

   a. Dietary intake:

      i. Eat a diet rich in calcium.

      ii. Eat a diet high in fiber.

      iii. Eat a diet with balanced macronutrients (calories from fat, carbohydrate, and protein in proportions for age recommended by Dietary Reference Intakes).

      iv. Encouragement, support, and maintenance of breastfeeding.

   b. Eating behaviors:

      i. Limiting consumption of energy-dense foods.

** Restrictive parenting (heavy monitoring and controlling of a child's behavior).

Physical Education Requirements by State

Alabama: Grades K–8 are required to take thirty minutes minimum per day; in high school, one year or two semesters are required.

Alaska: High schools require one unit of health and/or PE for graduation; other levels are determined by local school districts.

Arizona: PE is required in grades 1–8; high school requirements are decided by local school districts.

Arkansas: PE is mandated for grades K–12; the amount of time required varies by grade level.

California: PE is required in 100 percent of schools at all grade levels.

Colorado: Only 20 percent of high schools might have PE. Local school districts impose requirements; no statistics available for time requirements.

Connecticut: PE is mandated in every school curriculum. One hundred percent of schools provide PE at all levels; time requirements vary by grade level.

Delaware: No mandated PE in grades K–6; however, most schools provide thirty to sixty minutes per week. PE is mandated in grades 7–8.

District of Columbia: Ninety-five percent of lower grades have a PE program. Middle and high school levels are required to have a PE program.

Florida: No PE requirements for grades K–8; two semesters are mandated for the high school level.

Georgia: Grades K–6 have ninety hours of required PE. Grades 7–8 might have available classes but they are not mandatory. In high school, two classes are required and are usually completed in 9th grade.

Hawaii: Grades K–6 are expected to participate in PE; grades 7–12 must participate one year or two semesters.

Idaho: PE is required for grades 1–8; high schools are not required to offer physical education.

Illinois: State requires daily physical education grades K–12.

Indiana: PE is mandated at all levels as part of a larger program; two semesters are required to graduate from high school.

Iowa: PE is mandated for all grade levels; time requirements vary by grade level.

Kansas: PE is mandated by the state for grades K–6 and 9–12, but not for grades 7–8.

Kentucky: PE is mandated for all grade levels; time requirements vary by grade level.

Louisiana: PE is mandated for all grade levels; grades 9–12 must pass 270 hours of PE and 90 hours of health to graduate.

Maine: Grades K–6 and 9–12 have specific requirements; grades 7–8 requirements are determined by local school districts.

Maryland: PE is required by the state for all levels; each local school district provides a program.

Massachusetts: PE is required by the state for all levels; each local school district provides a program.

Michigan: PE is required by the state for all levels; each local school district provides a program.

Minnesota: PE is mandated by the state for all levels, but no times or specific grades are mentioned.

Mississippi: PE is mandated for grades K–8; it is not mandatory for high schools.

Missouri: PE is required by the state for all levels; it must be passed in high school to graduate.

Montana: Grades K–6 have daily PE requirements. Grades 7–8 have one semester per year required. Two semesters are required for grades 9–12.

Nebraska: Local school districts impose requirements; no statewide standards or fitness testing.

Nevada: PE is required only for high school; no statewide standards or fitness testing.

New Hampshire: All schools offer PE; local school boards determine time requirements.

New Jersey: Grades 1–12 must have 150 minutes of health, PE, and safety per week.

New Mexico: For grades K–6, students must meet standards from the state. One year of PE is required for grade 7. For grades 9–12, one year is required during the four.

New York: PE is required by the state for all levels; 120 minutes per week, every semester, is required.

North Carolina: PE is required for grades K–8, but they have no specific time requirements. One semester is required for grades 9–12.

North Dakota: PE is mandated for all grade levels; time requirements vary by grade level.

Ohio: Schools are required to teach PE as part of a total school program; local districts decide specific minutes per day or week that are required.

Oklahoma: School districts decide how to meet state PE standards.

Oregon: PE is required for all grade levels; one year of 130 hours is required for graduation from high school.

Pennsylvania: PE is mandated for all grade levels; time requirements vary by grade level.

Rhode Island: State requires 100 minutes of health and PE per week every year at all levels.

South Carolina: PE is required for all levels, but no specific minutes per week are required for grades K–8. Grades 9–12 must complete one semester of personal fitness and one semester of lifetime fitness.

South Dakota: No statewide requirements; local school districts determine requirements.

Tennessee: PE is required for grades K–8; grades 9–12 can take PE as an elective.

Texas: State requires that PE be offered to all students. Local school districts decide for grades K–8. Specific requirements are set for grades 9–12.

Utah: PE is required for all levels but times vary; some PE is required to graduate from high school.

Vermont: State requires 100 percent of schools at all levels offer PE. Grades K–8 have PE twice a week; grades 9–12 must have three semesters.

Virginia: State requires schools to provide PE for grades K–7. For grade 8, PE is one of four electives. Grades 9–12, two units of health and PE are required to graduate.

Washington: Grades K–8 are required to conduct PE classes for at least 100 minutes per week each year. High schools must offer PE for all four years.

West Virginia: PE is required for grades K–8 every year; grades 9–12 must complete one class.

Wisconsin: Grades K–6 must meet three times a week. Grades 7–8 meet a minimum of once a week. High schools require 1.5 credits for graduation.

Wyoming: State requires that 100 percent of schools at all levels offer PE; each local school district sets specific requirements.

---

* *Source:* Information courtesy of the National Association for Sport and Physical Education in Reston, Virginia; (800) 213-7193, ext. 410; www.aahperd.org/naspe.

APPENDIX C
Additional Resources

Organizations

The following organizations can answer questions and provide referrals to other information sources. Be aware that addresses and phone numbers are subject to change.

**American Academy of
  Pediatrics**
141 Northwest Point Blvd.
Elk Grove Village, IL 60007
(847) 434-4000
www.aap.org

American Heart Association
National Center
7272 Greenville Avenue
Dallas, TX 75231
(800) AHA-USA-1 (800-242-
  8721)
www.americanheart.org/presenter.
  jhtml?identifier=1200000

**Anorexia Nervosa and Related
  Eating Disorders (ANRED)**
P.O. Box 5102
Eugene, OR 97405
(503) 344-1144
www.anred.com

**Broda Barnes Research
  Foundation** (*for Hypothyroidism*)
P.O. Box 110098
Trumbull, CT 06611
(203) 261-2101
www.brodabarnes.org
(See also, *Hypothyroidism and
  Unsuspected Illness* by Broda
  Barnes, HarperCollins, 1976)

Centers for Disease Control (CDC) and Prevention
1600 Clifton Road
Atlanta, GA 30333
(404) 498-1515 or (800) 311-3435
www.cdc.gov

National Institutes of Health
9000 Rockville Pike
Bethesda, Maryland 20892
(301) 496-4000
www.nih.gov

Education Resources Information Center (ERIC)
c/o Computer Sciences Corporation
655 15th St. NW, Suite 500
Washington, DC 20005
800-LET-ERIC (800-538-3742)
www.eric.ed.gov

Websites

The following list of websites is provided for those who wish to do further research on the subject of childhood obesity. They are all excellent sources of vital information; however, this list is by no means complete. There are many other sources as well, and a keyword search under "childhood obesity" or related words will reveal these other sources. Be aware that there are many "blogs" on the Internet that have less credibility than sources whose content is written and reviewed by others in their respective professions. There are also web-based sources whose primary aim is to promote a specific weight-loss or home-exercise product or product line. The sources that can be considered the most reliable are those that are written by, and peer-reviewed by, those in the medical, physical education, nutrition, and related professions. Be aware, also, that web addresses are subject to change.

Health Day News: www.healthday.com

Inch-Aweigh: www.inch-aweigh.com

Kid Source: www.kidsource.com

Kids' Games: www.gameskidsplay.net

Kids' Health: www.kidshealth.org

Mayo Clinic: www.mayoclinic.com

Medscape: www.medscape.com

NYU Child Study Center: www.aboutourkids.org

WebMD: www.WebMD.com

Bibliography

Chapter 1

Apple Products Research & Education Council. "Parents Confuse Fruit 'Drinks' with the Real Thing." *HealthSource Online*, July 27, 1998. www.kidsource.com/kidsource/content4/fruit.juice.news.html

Belluck, Pam. "Obesity and High Cholesterol in Children Are Seen as Warning of Heart Disease." *New York Times*, Nov 12, 2008: www.nytimes.com/2008/11/12/health/12heart.html?_r=1&sq=Obesity%20and%20High%20Cholesterol%20in%20Children%20Are%20Seen%20as%20Warning%20of%20Heart%20Disease&st=nyt&oref=slogin&scp=2&pagewanted=print (accessed Nov 14, 2008)

Boys and Girls Clubs of America Report. "Youth Trends: An Environmental Scan in Support of Impact 2012," 2008

DeNoon, Daniel. "1 in 3 American Teens Unfit." *WebMD*, Oct 2, 2006. www.webmd.com/content/article/128/116961?printing=true (accessed Oct 3, 2006)

Goodman, Robin F. "Developing Healthy Eating Behaviors in Children." *AboutOurKids.org*. www.aboutourkids.org/articles/developing_healthy_eating_behaviors (undated, accessed Feb 27, 2008)

Hitti, Miranda. "As Kids' TV Time Rises, Grades Fall." *WebMD*, Oct 2, 2006. www.webmd.com/content/article/128/116962?printing=true (accessed Oct 3, 2006)

Hitti, Miranda. "Overweight Tots Apt to Stay Fat." *WebMD*, Sept 5, 2006. www.webmd.com/content/Article/127/116562.htm (accessed Sept 13, 2006)

National Institute of Diabetes & Digestive & Kidney Diseases. Weight-control Information Network. "Helping Your Overweight Child." www.niddk.nih.gov (undated, accessed Feb 27, 2008)

Pallarito, Karen. "Childhood Obesity a Long-Term Challenge." *HealthDay*, Sept 20, 2007. http://news.aol.com/story/_a/childhood-obesity-epidemic-a-long-term/n20070920170809990011 (accessed Dec 19, 2007)

Sack, Kevin. "Schools Found Improving on Nutrition and Fitness." *New York Times*, Oct 20, 2007, A9

Uranga, Rachel. "Obesity Among Children Grows More Problematic." *Times-Picayune* (New Orleans, LA), May 8, 2005, A36 (previously published in *Los Angeles Daily News*)

Chapter 2

Georgetown Center for Food and Nutrition Policy. "Top Pediatricians and Nutrition Policy Experts Say Exercise and a Balanced Diet Are Best Tools to Fight Childhood Obesity." www.kidsource.com/health/fight.child.obesity.html, Feb 24, 2000.

Hitti, Miranda. "Pediatricians: Kids Vulnerable to Ads." *WebMD*, Dec 4, 2006. www.webmd.com/content/article/130/117695?printing=true (accessed Dec 6, 2006).

Mozes, Alan. "Obesity-Linked Woes Boost Kids' Lifetime Heart Risk. *HealthDay News*, Mar 23, 2008. http://abcnews.go.com/Health/Healthday/Story?id=4508259&page=1 (accessed Oct. 22, 2008)

Paddock, Catharine. "Obesity Gene Discovered." *Medical News Today* online, Apr 13, 2007. www.medicalnewstoday.com/articles/67666.php

Shaibi, Gabriel, Christian Roberts, and Michael Goran. "Exercise and Insulin Resistance in Youth." *Journal of American College of Sports Medicine*, Jan 2008; 36(1). www.medscape.com/viewarticle/568391_print (accessed Feb 18, 2008)

Stubbe, Janine H., Dorret I. Boomsma, and Eco J.C. de Geus, "Sports Participation During Adolescence: A Shift from Environmental to Genetic Factors." *Medicine and Science in Sports and Exercise*, Nov 2005; 37(4): 563–570

Ukkola, Olavi and Claude Bouchard. "Genetic Factors and Childhood Obesity." Report of the Nestlé Nutrition Workshop, Obesity in Childhood and in Adolescence, Shanghai, China, Apr 22–26, 2001. *Annales Nestle*, 59: 59–68

Virtua Health. "Managing Obesity and Cholesterol in Kids." *Kidsource*, July 24, 2001. www.kidsource.com/health/control.cholest.html (accessed Oct 22, 2008)

Wilbert, Caroline. "Study Shows Physical Activity Can Offset Genetic Predisposition for Obesity." *WebMD Health News*, Sept 8, 2008. www.medicinenet.com/script/main/art.asp?articlekey=92509

Chapter 3

American Medical Association. "Expert Committee Recommendations on the Assessment, Prevention, and Treatment of Child and Adolescent Overweight and Obesity." Jan 25, 2007. www.ama-assn.org/ama1/pub/upload/mm/433/ped_obesity_recs.pdf

"Body Fat Percentage Calculator." *Inch-Aweigh.com*. www.inch-aweigh.com/calc_body_fat.htm (accessed Feb 25, 2008)

Boyles, Salynn. "Childhood Diabetes Ups Kidney Risk." *WebMD*, July 25, 2006. www.webmd.com/content/Article/125/116018.htm (accessed July 27, 2006)

Boyles, Salynn. "Kids with Diabetes Face Heart Risks." *WebMD*, Jul 27, 2006. www.webmd.com/content/Article/125/116059.htm (accessed August 16, 2006)

Children's Hospital of Philadelphia. "Obesity," Jul 20, 2003. www.chop.edu/consumer/your_child/condition_section_index.jsp?id=9422&printable

Hellmich, Nanci. "Why Are Parents in Denial About Kids' Weight?" *USA Today* online, Sept 3, 2007. http://usatoday.com/news/health/2007-09-03-overweight-kids_N.htm?POE=clickrefer (accessed Sept. 12, 2007)

"Hemoglobin A1c (HbA1c) Test for Diabetes." *WebMD*, Mar 23, 2005. http://diabetes. webmd.com/guide/glycated-hemoglobin-test-hba1c (accessed Feb 25, 2008)

Quinn, Elizabeth. "Body Composition: Body Fat, Body Weight." *About.com: Sports Medicine*, updated Mar 17, 2008. http://sportsmedicine.about.com/od/fitnessevalandassessment/a/Body_Fat_Comp.htm (accessed Oct 22, 2008)

Revolution Health Group. "Project PACT—Parents and Children Fighting Obesity." www.revolutionhealth.com/healthy-living/weight-management/special-feature/childhood-obesity (accessed Feb 25, 2008)

Sulemana, Habiba, Michael Smolensky, and Dejian Lai. "Relationship Between Physical Activity and Body Mass Index in Adolescents." *Medicine & Science in Sports & Exercise*, Jun 2006; 38(6): 1182–1186

Chapter 4

Hitti, Miranda. "Extreme Obesity in Tots Tied to Low IQ." *WebMD*, Aug 31, 2006. www.webmd.com/content/Article/126/116539.htm (accessed Sept 13, 2006)

Warner, Jennifer. "Overweight Girls Suffer at School." *WebMD*, Sept 8, 2006. www.webmd.com/content/Article/127/116625.htm (accessed Sept 11, 2006)

Chapter 5

Boyles, Salynn. "Childhood Diabetes Ups Kidney Risk." *WebMD*, Jul 25, 2006. www.webmd.com/content/Article/125/116018.htm (accessed Jul 27, 2006)

Boyles, Salynn. "Kids with Diabetes Face Heart Risks." *WebMD*, Jul 27, 2006. www.webmd.com/content/Article/125/116059.htm (accessed Aug 16, 2006)

Boyles, Salynn. "Just for Teens' Cholesterol Analysis." *WebMD*, Aug 29, 2006. www.webmd.com/content/Article/125/116512.htm (accessed Sept 11, 2006)

Gordon, Serena. "Food Restrictions on Kids Backfire." *HealthDayNews*, Oct 4, 2007. Reprinted on SingleMom.com (www.singlemom.com/HealthAndWellBeing/sg_Study_Food_Restrictions_on_Kids_Backfire.aspx)

Hellmich, Nanci. "Why Are Parents in Denial about Kids' Weight?" *USA Today* online, Sept 3, 2007. www.usatoday.com/news/health/2007-09-03-overweight-kids_N.htm?POE=click-refer (Sept 3, 2007)

Hitti, Miranda. "Obesity, Heart Disease May Start Young." *WebMD* Medical News, Jan 8, 2007. www.webmd.com/content/Article/131/117992.htm (accessed Jan 9, 2007)

Hitti, Miranda. "Pediatricians: Kids Vulnerable to Ads." *WebMD*, Dec 4, 2006. www.webmd.com/content/Article/130/117695.htm (accessed Dec 6, 2006)

International Food Information Council Foundation and Council of Better Business Bureaus. "A Practical Guide to Parents: Advertising, Nutrition and Kids." 1993. Reprinted on *KidSource Online*. www.kidsource.com/kidsource/pages/health.nutrition.html

International Food Information Council Foundation. "Sizing Up Kids' Nutrition and Fitness." Undated. Reprinted on *KidSource Online*. www.kidsource.com/kidsource/pages/health.nutrition.html

National Institute of Diabetes & Digestive & Kidney Diseases. Weight-control Information Network. "Helping Your Overweight Child." Undated. http://win.niddk.nih.gov/publications/over_child.htm

Processed Apples Institute. "Parents Confuse Fruit 'Drinks' with the Real Thing," July 27, 1998. www.applejuice.org

"Schools Need to Help Fight Obesity." *Times-Picayune*, New Orleans, LA (from *HealthDay News*), Oct 16, 2004

Summerfield, Liane M. "Childhood Obesity." *ERIC Digest*, Dec 1990; ED328556

Chapter 7

American Medical Association. "Expert Committee Recommendations on the Assessment, Prevention, and Treatment of Child and Adolescent Overweight and Obesity." Jan 25, 2007. www.ama-assn.org/ama1/pub/upload/mm/433/ped_obesity_recs.pdf

DeNoon, Daniel. "1 in 3 American Teens Unfit." *WebMD*, Oct 2, 2006. www.webmd.com/content/Article/128/116961.htm (accessed Oct 3, 2006)

Educational Research and Improvement Clearinghouse (ERIC). "Childhood Obesity." *ERIC Digest*, 1990; ED 328556

Fries, Wendy C. "Encouraging Exercise in Your Kids." *WebMD*, Oct 25, 2004, updated Aug 16, 2006. www.webmd.com//content/Article/95/103524.htm (accessed Sept 11, 2006)

Kendall, P, K. Wilken, and E. Serrano. Colorado State University Extension, Nutrition Resources. "Childhood Obesity." Article #9.317 (undated). www.ext.colostate.edu/pubs/foodnut/09317.html

Napoli, MaryAnn. "The Bogalusa Heart Study of 14,000 Children." *HealthFacts*, Aug 1, 1998. http://findarticles.com/p/articles/mi_m0815/is_n8_v23/ai_21155460

Stelter, Brian. "Report Ties Children's Use of Media to Their Health. *New York Times*, Dec 1, 2008. www.nytimes.com/2008/12/02/arts/02stud.html?_r=1&scp=1&sq=report+ties+children%27s+use+of+media+to+their+health&st=nyt

Tulane University Medical Center School of Public Health and Tropic Medicine Center for Cardiovascular Health. "The Bogalusa Heart Study." www.som.tulane.edu/cardiohealth/bog.html

Chapter 8

Henig, Robin Marantz. "Why Do We Play?" *New York Times Magazine*, Feb 17, 2008

Chapter 9

Kids' Games. Updated Jan 28, 2007. www.gameskidsplay.net (accessed Mar 31, 2008)

Index

About the Author

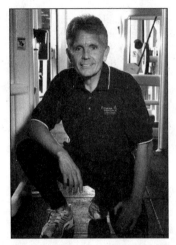

Mackie Shilstone is one of America's most influential sports performance managers, whose expertise has played a pivotal role in the success and longevity of more than 3,000 professional athletes. His clients have included tennis star Serena Williams; baseball Hall of Famer Ozzie Smith; former world champion boxers, Michael Spinks, Riddick Bowe, Roy Jones Jr., and Bernard Hopkins; and all-time leading NFL scorer Morten Andersen.

With a Master of Arts degree and Master of Business Administration, Mackie currently directs The Fitness Principle with Mackie Shilstone at East Jefferson General Hospital in Metairie, Louisiana. He is the author of five previous books, *Lean & Hard* (John Wiley & Sons, 2007), *The Fat-Burning Bible* (John Wiley & Sons, 2005), *Maximum Energy for Life* (John Wiley & Sons, 2003), *Lose Your Love Handles* (Perigee, 2001), and *Feelin' Good About Fitness* (Pelican Publishing, 1986). Mackie has also written articles for prestigious health and fitness journals, including the *American Medical Athletic Association Quarterly* and *The Physiologist.*

Additionally, Mackie is a clinical instructor of public health and preventative medicine at Louisiana State Health Sciences Center, adjunct professor at the A. B. Freeman School of Business at Tulane University, and special advisor to the U.S. Olympic Committee on Sports Nutrition. He has served on the Governor's Council on Physical Fitness and Sports, State of Louisiana.

Mackie's innovative approaches to sports training have been reported in over 2,000 newspaper and magazine articles, including *The Wall Street Journal, The New York Times, Los Angeles Times, USA Today, Inc.* and *People* magazine. *KO Magazine* voted him among the top fifty most influential people in the history of boxing. He has also appeared on most of the major news shows in the U.S., including *ESPN,* the *Today* show, Fox News Channel, HBO, *48 Hours, Live with Regis and Kelly,* and *Good Morning America.*

Mackie, a regular on local TV and contributor to area publications, lives in New Orleans with his wife, Sandra, and their two sons, Spencer and Scott.